Facing Cancer With God's Help

A Personal Journey

Jeanne Carol Martin

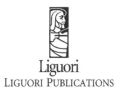

Liguori

LIGUORI PUBLICATIONS

Imprimi Potest:
Harry Grile, CSsR, Provincial
Denver Province, The Redemptorists

Published by Liguori Publications
Liguori, Missouri 63057

To order, visit Liguori.org or call 800-325-9521.

Library of Congress Cataloging-in-Publication Data

Martin, Jeanne Carol.
 Facing cancer with God's help : a personal journey / Jeanne Carol Martin
 —Memorial Edition.
 pages cm

1. Martin, Jeanne Carol. 2. Cancer—Patients—Religious life. 3. Cancer—
 Patients—Biography. 4. Catholics—Religious life. I. Title.
 BV4910.33.M37 2014
 248.8'61969940092—dc23
 2014031280

p ISBN: 978-0-7648-2491-3
e ISBN: 978-0-7648-6937-2

Liguori Publications, a nonprofit corporation, is an apostolate of
The Redemptorists. To learn more about The Redemptorists, visit
Redemptorists.com.

Printed in the United States of America
18 17 16 15 14 / 5 4 3 2 1
First Edition

Contents

❧

Dedicated to
Our Mother of Perpetual Help

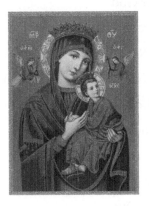

For surely I know the plans
I have for you, says the LORD,
plans for your welfare
and not for harm, to give you
a future with hope.

JEREMIAH 29:11

ৡৡ

Prologue

❧

*M*ay 5, 1998; Tuesday. I checked my voice
mail after the last school bell at 3:00 p.m.
This tiny closet with a faculty phone gave perfect
privacy from the commotion in the hallway at
dismissal. I didn't know what to think when I
heard Dr. Denes had called and wanted to talk to
me about the results of my CT scan on Saturday.
Let's see...if it was bad news, wouldn't he call by
Monday evening? But if it was good news, wouldn't
his nurse just leave a message at home? They called
me at school. I usually get the calls about my tests
at home. Did this mean it was bad news? I was
barely breathing as my fingers stumbled through
the numbers to call his office. When I asked for him,
they put me right through. Now I knew something
was wrong. Usually they would say he was seeing
patients and would call back at the end of the day.
I felt frozen. I had been clear for eighteen months.
No sign of recurrence of my kidney cancer when I
had the last scan five months ago. Then Dr. Denes
came on the line. I didn't hear clearly past his first
words telling me there was a spot on my remaining
kidney again. A warm flush came over my entire

*body. My stomach fell. Tears welled up. I began
biting my lip to keep from becoming hysterical. I
wanted to scream. No, it can't be. I've been doing
everything right. I'm a good person. I go to church,
talk to God, love my family. I've read Bernie Siegel,
and I meditate and exercise and eat right. There
must be some mistake. I deserve to live. I've been
clear for eighteen months. The radiologist must not
know how to read my scans. They are difficult because of the scar tissue from the last surgery. Stop. I
couldn't comprehend what he was saying. What? A
tumor on a lymph node in my right chest? Say that
again. Stop! What small nodules in my lungs? You
never told me about that. They've been there for a
year? My God, I must be dreaming. Surely, this is
just a bad dream...a nightmare. I could barely talk
in between the sobs and trying to take in some air.
Carrie, our oldest daughter, is getting married in a
few weeks. I can't do this to her and to my family
again. I don't have any fight left. How am I going
to get through this again?*

ॐ

This was just one day in my ongoing battle with
cancer, facing the same question all cancer patients face:
"How am I going to get through this?" When I seemed
to have my cancer under control, I envisioned writing
a book about what steps cancer patients should take
when they are diagnosed. Then on June 15, 2000, my
scans showed new tumors around my pancreas and yet

another in my kidney, plus growth of the existing tumors that I thought were stable. At that diagnosis, I realized two important truths. One is that I do not have the key to conquering cancer. The other major realization is that I feel a deep sense of peace with this seventh diagnosis of new tumors that I had not felt before. So my recurring question, "How am I going to get through this?" is finding an answer: "With God's help!" I feel God's presence in my life in such a profound and intimate way that I can say, "It's OK." God is walking with me on this journey, and I may be led to a cure, and if not, then God will be by my side and with my family to accept dying.

Then came the dreaded phone calls. I had to call my married daughter to tell her of my new tumors. She exploded, "How can you believe in a God who would do this to you?" Then I knew that I wanted to write about how God has helped me through my struggle with cancer and not caused my cancer. The following chapters detail my "God connection." I share my very real and personal story of my close encounter with God that resulted in replacing my fear, anxiety, depression, and hopelessness with courage, peace, joy, and hope. Many people ask me how I do it—how I seem so positive, happy, peaceful. This book is my story of how God has made a difference in my life as I face living with cancer. This book is written to give hope and a sense of peace to others in the race for good health. I am also writing to leave a legacy to my children on how faith and God played a key role in my cancer battle.

Teaching high-school theology classes, adult Bible studies, Christian-initiation programs, and receiving a master's degree in religious studies have prepared me well to know to reach for God when I am down and out. But knowing about God is only the beginning. Experiencing God's presence in my heart is on a completely different level. And that is where my cancer diagnosis has taken me—on a heart-to-heart journey with Jesus.

My cancer history is recurrent renal cell carcinoma (kidney cancer). I was first diagnosed in 1984, at age thirty-five. My right kidney was removed. In 1986, the cancer had metastasized to my right ovary, resulting in a hysterectomy. In 1996, I underwent three surgeries to remove metastatic kidney tumors from my left chest, thyroid, and left kidney. Since neither chemotherapy nor radiation is effective in treating kidney cancer, surgery has been my only option.

After my three surgeries in 1996, I was afraid my body was a time bomb ready to go off again. This period marked the beginning of my research to help myself prevent a recurrence. This turmoil also initiated a deepening of my friendship with God. The next two years were spent researching the mind/body/spirit connection with wellness, and choosing tools that I thought would help me (for example, meditation, visualization, healing touch, prayer, tai chi). Unfortunately, I found I still had a lot to learn.

My CT scan on May 2, 1998, showed that multiple tumors had recurred—nodules in both lungs, spots on my left kidney, and a tumor in my right chest. Surgery was no longer an option since I would risk losing a lung due to the positioning of the tumor. I was also at risk of losing my left kidney since it had already been resectioned (that is, previously operated on to remove tumors). If operated on, I would possibly have only one lung, be on dialysis, and still be at risk for more cancer spread. After choosing alternative treatments and being relatively stable for two years, my scans on June 15, 2000, showed three new tumors around my pancreas, a new tumor in my kidney, and growth of the chest tumor. I have gradually grown in my relationship with God, and I feel God empowering me each day to embrace life and live it to the fullest.

By sharing my story, it is my hope that others with cancer or life-threatening illnesses will discover a deeper connection with God that provides the comfort, encouragement, and peace desired and needed for this journey. It is also my sincere hope that these chapters will be read by family and friends of those with serious illness in order to better understand our inner struggle with life-and-death issues and the priceless value of a strong and growing faith perspective. Family and friends play a pivotal role. God's love is certainly made real through their caring, support, and prayers.

ૐ

God has two dwellings. One in heaven and the other in the...thankful heart.

IZAAK WALTON (1593–1683)

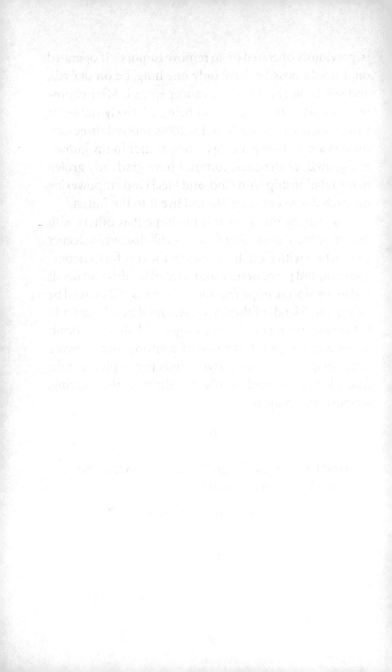

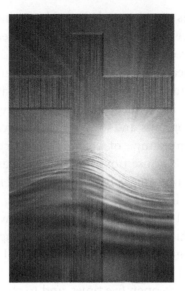

– Chapter One –

Reaching for God

❧

Reaching for God
He did not say,
"You will not be troubled;
you will not be labored;
you will not be afflicted."
But he did say,
"You will not be overcome."

JULIAN OF NORWICH (C. 1342–C. 1420)

Earlier this year, I attended a leader training meeting at a cancer support center. I volunteered to present a program from a cancer survivor's viewpoint on what to expect, ideas on the need for support after a cancer diagnosis, and personal insights about what helped me through my cancer recurrences. Included with a list of therapies, programs, and stress reduction techniques was my faith as an example of what helped me cope with my cancer. The response from the director was to caution me about mentioning faith. He said it could make people uncomfortable.

My initial response was to agree, but inwardly I soon questioned his reasoning. It was by turning to God for support and guidance that I was able to find the strength and courage I needed to face the unknown, to allow surgeons to cut me open five times, and to choose difficult treatment options. My faith was the most important tool I had, and now I was not supposed to mention it? Turning to God is a significant part of my cancer experience. To ignore that dimension when I am sharing my cancer experience would be a lie. I am not really talking about "me," if I hide the part about God.

My experience with many cancer patients over the last four years tells me that the God connection is a common denominator. When we feel hopeless and helpless, we want to believe there is a higher power out there who is in control. Inviting God to be a part of our cancer situation is normal, natural, and healthy.

Bringing a faith perspective to our illness can result in replacing fear and anxiety with the peace and joy for living each day. A God connection can bring meaning and acceptance to our suffering and can allow us to understand the good that is possible even in the face of cancer.

People often tell me that they admire my strength and courage. They comment on my calm nature and the happiness that is reflected in my smile. I do go about living each day, not as a cancer fighter, but as a person welcoming the gifts of each new day. This person just happens to have cancer. The source of this inner strength and peace is my faith, my connection with God, which has evolved and deepened as I have experienced the ups and downs of living with cancer. Because it is alive, my faith will continue to grow and change. Dependence on God is not a sign of weakness but a natural response to the love God has for me.

The first thing God helped me with after my May 1998 recurrence of inoperable tumors was the decision to fight. I was feeling incredible panic, fear, and anxiety for the future. When I looked in the mirror, I wondered how long I would have left to live. This was an important time for our family. We had a daughter getting married, a daughter graduating from college, and our youngest daughter graduating from high school. And here I was, drawing a black cloud over all the good things that were happening to us.

I thought about my fight of the last fourteen years and five surgeries. There was a flicker of a thought that said, "What will be, will be. I'm tired of fighting. Maybe it's time to give in and give up. Haven't I put my family through enough heartache? Maybe they would be better off without me." I realized that I had not really made the decision to fight. Rather, I was going along with what was expected of me. I knew it would take more courage on my part to fight than to give up. I remembered reading about the importance and power of the will to live. And I whispered a simple prayer, "Oh, God, help me." And I began to see that I was not alone. I had a husband of twenty-five years and three daughters who would be my personal cheerleaders. I had four sisters who would go to the ends of the earth to help and support me. Most of all, I had God walking by my side. I would turn this diagnosis into the beginning of an adventure, not a certain death sentence.

I was on a journey that would take me to places in my heart and mind that I had not visited before. I would be faced with opportunities that challenged me to grow.

❧

Do not let your hearts be troubled.
Believe in God, believe also in me.

JOHN 14:1

Come to me, all you that are weary and are carrying heavy burdens, and I will give you rest. Take my yoke upon you, and learn from me; for I am gentle and humble in heart, and you will find rest for your souls. For my yoke is easy, and my burden is light.

MATTHEW 11:28–30

Dear God,
At times, I feel so afraid, lonely, and anxious.
I don't want to die. I'm afraid of what lies ahead
for myself and my family. Please take my hand
and lead me to a deeper connection with your
ever-present love for me. Help me to believe in
your presence in my life, and walk with me on
this journey with cancer.
Amen.

ॐ

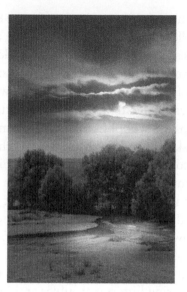

– Chapter Two –

Healing Through the Eucharist

ℬ

Jesus said to them, "I am the bread of life.
Whoever comes to me will never be hungry,
and whoever believes in me will never be thirsty."

JOHN 6:35

One morning, I was running late for the 8 a.m. Mass, and pulled into the parking lot to see about twice as many cars as usual for a Tuesday. I wondered if I had forgotten some special feast day. By the time I parked and got out of the car, I had decided that it was a normal weekday morning. I had no idea why the extra cars were there. Perhaps the school had early parent meetings. As I walked briskly toward the back door of church, I met another latecomer. I smiled a greeting and said off-handedly, "They must be giving something away today."

I zipped into church, and took a back pew just in time to hear the homily. Then it hit me. They are "giving something away" in here—Jesus, himself. Each of us sitting quietly in our pews, all spaced apart for personal devotion, were in church for the purpose of receiving Jesus, and to bring him our troubles and joys. We were at Mass to receive our free gift—the person of Jesus in holy Communion. If all those people sitting in rush-hour traffic outside really understood what was taking place in here, the church would be packed. Here I was, day after day, conscious of the wonderful gift I was receiving. The Eucharist, Jesus' Body and Blood, offers me hope, healing, strength, courage, and peace. And it's free to all who come.

I had come to Mass that day to beg and plead with God to help me with my cancer recurrence. The Gospel that day was the story of the woman with a hemorrhage. Jesus was traveling with the disciples to a synagogue leader's house to attend to his little girl who was ill.

> Now there was a woman who had been suffering from hemorrhages for twelve years. She had

endured much under many physicians, and had spent all that she had; and she was no better, but rather grew worse. She had heard about Jesus, and came up behind him in the crowd and touched his cloak, for she said, "If I but touch his clothes, I will be made well." Immediately her hemorrhage stopped; and she felt in her body that she was healed of her disease. Immediately aware that power had gone forth from him, Jesus turned about in the crowd and said, "Who touched my clothes?"

And his disciples said to him, "You see the crowd pressing in on you; how can you say, 'Who touched me?'"

He looked all around to see who had done it. But the woman, knowing what had happened to her, came in fear and trembling, fell down before him, and told him the whole truth. He said to her, "Daughter, your faith has made you well; go in peace, and be healed of your disease."

MARK 5:25–34

I immediately identified with this poor woman. It had been twelve years since my original diagnosis of kidney cancer in 1984. The woman in the Scripture was afflicted for twelve years and had no healing from the doctors. I, too, had consulted many doctors since my original diagnosis. She longed to touch Jesus' cloak to be cured. I was here at Mass, longing to touch Jesus and be healed. As I followed the people in line for Communion, I pictured myself being just like the woman with the hemorrhage, inching herself through the crowd in order to reach Jesus. This was even better than touching Jesus' cloak. I was actually touching Jesus, himself. I raised my hands as the priest offered me the Body of Christ. "Amen., I believe." As I took the host, I knew Jesus was as close to me as the woman who saw Jesus face to face. The power and gift of the Eucharist overwhelmed me.

My personal treatment plan includes daily Mass. It is equally as important as nutrition, supplements, exercise, or immune therapy. However, this component treats more than my cancer. Receiving Jesus in the Eucharist heals my soul, my spirit, and my mind. I believe that each time I receive Communion, Jesus takes my physical and emotional pain and allows me to be free of the burden. "He took our infirmities and bore our diseases" (Matthew 8:17). As Jesus becomes a part of me, my thoughts turn to wondering how anything harmful, like cancer, could possibly live in a vessel filled with holiness and God himself. And I am filled with hope.

At Mass, I listen to the Word of God proclaimed in the Scriptures, and allow God to touch my heart. The prayers speak to my brokenness and humility. "Lord, have mercy on me." I join my prayers with those who share their brokenness and need for healing during the petitions. There is someone with lupus, a man whose spouse has cancer, another person has just been diagnosed with multiple sclerosis. A woman behind me just lost her husband, a man across the aisle lost his job, someone's grandchild is sick, another has a son who left home. We are all broken and come to the table of the Lord to be touched and healed. I am not alone.

The Eucharist celebrates Jesus' victory over death. "Dying you destroyed our death, rising you restored our life. Lord Jesus, come in glory." I need to hear that death is not the end. I need to know that my life will go on. The Eucharist reminds me that Jesus, too, suffered and died an early death. No matter how deep my suffering, I know that with Jesus' help I can experience a part of his rising.

"Lord, I am not worthy to receive you, but only say the word and I shall be healed." This is my prayer as I receive Jesus. I pray that I will be healed of my weaknesses, my sins, and my cancer. As I wait my turn in the line for Communion, I pray the prayer *Anima Christi.*

> Soul of Christ, sanctify me.
> Body of Christ, save me.
> Blood of Christ, inebriate me
> ["give me joy for living each day"].
> Water from the side of Christ, wash me
> ["wash me clean of my weaknesses and cancer"].
> Passion of Christ, strengthen me
> ["to fight this battle"].
> Good Jesus, hear me.
> Within your wounds hide me.
> Never permit me to be separated from you.
> From the evil one protect me.
> At the hour of my death,
>   call me and bid me come to you.
> That with your saints I may praise you
>   forever and ever.
> Amen.

I sit quietly and reverently with my eyes closed after Communion. I imagine and pray that the Body and Blood of Jesus will become one with my body and blood. I pray that it is Jesus' blood that beats through my heart, bringing wholeness and healing to all my good cells. I pray that Jesus will prevent any blood supply from reaching the cancer cells. I picture the blood flow throughout my body, in all my veins and arteries, having healing power because it is Jesus' divine blood. This is a healing visualization that makes sense to me, scientifically and spiritually.

The Mass is my refuge. It is the memorial of Jesus' death. I am welcomed to come and eat, and to take the body of Jesus that has been given up for me. I am invited to come and drink and take the blood of Jesus that was shed for me so that my sins may be forgiven. Jesus loved me so much that he gave his life for me. That compassionate divine love is extended to me each day through the Eucharist, the Real Presence of Jesus.

❧

"I am the bread of life. Your ancestors ate the manna in the wilderness, and they died. This is the bread that comes down from heaven, so that one may eat of it and not die. I am the living bread that came down from heaven. Whoever eats of this bread will live forever; and the bread that I will give for the life of the world is my flesh."

JOHN 6:48–51

Lord Jesus Christ,
Thank you for being present to me today
just as you were present to your apostles
and disciples two thousand years ago.
Oh Lord, when I am hurting and broken,
I need your healing touch to comfort me
and heal me. I come to you in the Eucharist to
receive your Body and Blood. I pray that your
Body and Blood become a part of my body,
strengthening me in my fight against cancer,
bringing me peace and comfort, and healing me
of my disease.
Amen.

❧

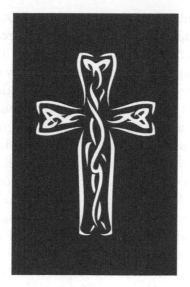

– Chapter Three –

God's Love Relieves Our Misery

ॐ

Commit your way to the LORD;
trust in him, and he will act.

PSALM 37:5

I was recently asked to give a presentation at a high-school senior retreat. The story I shared with the students was from my cancer journey and included my understanding of God's mercy as well as my call to trust God in this process of life with all its struggles and joys. This different way of looking at mercy, and my call to trust God, has had a profound effect not only on my relationship with God and my way of praying, but also on my sense of peace with life events, as well as trusting and believing God will take care of my concerns.

After my May 1998 diagnosis of inoperable tumors, I was caught up in a panic to find something that would help me survive. My oncologist had told me that no chemotherapy or radiation was known to be successful against kidney cancer. My five previous surgeries had been my lifeline. No more. The statistics gave me less than a five percent chance of surviving five years. My husband and I were busy with family activities. Luckily, planning a wedding that summer kept me from jumping into a treatment prematurely. My family used the time to research clinical trials and nutritional clinics, and to pray.

A week or so before our daughter's wedding, a woman from our parish approached me and told me to call her for some important information. That began a process of looking into an alternative cancer treatment that is located in Freeport, Bahamas. This immune-system treatment, founded by a New York researcher, has been in existence for twenty years and has no side effects. It works best on people without chemotherapy. I talked with a woman with kidney cancer who had been given a few months to live, her cancer having spread to her liver and throughout her abdomen. She had been getting treatment for nineteen years at the Bahama clinic. I regained hope. We flew to the Bahamas five days after our daughter's wedding.

So, there I was, in a strange country, being told I would have to stay for treatment for ten to twelve weeks. The treatment called for me to give myself injections up to twelve times a day. I had never before given myself one shot, much less twelve in one day. I hated needles. My husband's job required him to return home after the first two weeks. I had two days alone before our youngest daughter arrived to be my companion. Although I acted very strong in front of my husband as he was preparing to leave me, inside I was frightened—frightened to think about giving myself injections for the rest of my life, frightened that the treatment wouldn't work for me, frightened to be in a strange country, not knowing when I would return home. Was I crazy to be doing this? Would I end up dying anyway? I cried all the way back to my apartment after saying goodbye to my husband at the airport.

I walked out on the apartment terrace that night. The view was extraordinary. I sat in my chair on the verge of tears. This was a real low point in my life. I had packed some little prayer booklets from my night stand at home, and took one out on the balcony to read. I don't know who gave me the booklet, *The Divine Mercy Message and Devotion*[1]. I had never read it before, but it was the one I took to read on the terrace, and I am so grateful to the person who passed it on to me.

_____

1. Fr. Seraphim Michalenko, MIC, The Divine Mercy Message and Devotion (Stockbridge, MA: Marian Helpers, 1995)

The booklet described the story of a young woman named Helen, a member of the Sisters of Mercy, who lived in Poland and worked with troubled teens. She took the name Faustina when she entered the order. She was born the same year as my dad, 1905. When she was in her mid-twenties, she began having mystical experiences of Jesus speaking to her. She died at the age of thirty-three, leaving a large mystical legacy. Pope John Paul II validated the experiences and writings of Sister Faustina Kowalska when he canonized her in April 2000. There are three main parts to the message Jesus gave to her: Ask for and accept God's mercy, trust Jesus completely, and be merciful to others.

Here I was, looking out at the ocean with a horizon of dark blue sky, and I felt like this was God's message to me. I had always thought of "mercy" as pity—feeling sorry for someone. When I would say, "God have mercy on me," it implied, "forgive my sins and mistakes, and don't punish me as I deserve." I likened it to asking my parents to have mercy on me when they caught me coming in after curfew when I was a teenager, and of not wanting to be grounded. Jesus, however, told Faustina that mercy is love that seeks to relieve misery: Mercy is love in action! Mercy is nothing like my understanding of it had been.

With this new meaning of mercy, when I said, "Jesus have mercy on me," I was now asking Jesus to take away my misery—my fear of dying, of trying a new treatment, of being away from home for the summer. I felt broken and weak and *alone*, but I heard in this message of mercy that Jesus loved me so much, despite my sins, and wanted to do *something*—not just pity me or "refrain from punishing" me. Jesus wanted to give me his *mercy*—his *love*—and take away my misery. It was like getting a hug from Jesus.

Faustina quotes Jesus as saying:

Souls that make an appeal to my mercy delight me.
To such souls I grant even more than they ask.
I cannot punish even the greatest sinner
if he makes an appeal to my compassion.
No soul that has called upon my mercy has
ever been disappointed.[2]

I am love and mercy itself. Let no one fear to
draw near to me. My mercy is greater than your
sins and those of the entire world. I let my
Sacred Heart be pierced with a lance, thus
opening wide the source of mercy for you.
Come then with trust to draw graces from this
fountain.[3]

The second part of Jesus' message treats asking for—and accepting—God's mercy. If I was asking for God to relieve my misery and help me, then I had to completely trust Jesus to do it his way. I had to let go of my preconceived ideas of what is best for me. My ideas included a miraculous healing of my cancer, spontaneous remission, and so on. I realized that to truly trust meant that I might die. But if I believed Jesus loved me so much and wanted to relieve my misery, then I had to trust that he was in

---

2 *op. cit.*, page 24

3 *ibid.*, page 27

control. Jesus told Faustina, "I have opened my heart as a living fountain of mercy. Let all souls draw life from it. Let them approach this sea of mercy with trust. The graces of my mercy are drawn by means of one vessel only, and that is...trust. The more a soul trusts, the more it will receive."[4]

I began a new relationship with Jesus that night. I told him, on the terrace overlooking the ocean, with the stars coming out and the moon shining on the water, that I trusted him with my life—my journey— whether I would live or die and whatever might lie between. "Jesus, I trust in you," I said.

The third part of Jesus' message to Faustina was to be merciful—to love others and seek to relieve their misery. I realized that often I don't see someone else's misery because I'm so self-absorbed. Nothing can make you more self-absorbed than having cancer! I often expected our household decisions to revolve around me and my wants and needs.

Faustina writes of Jesus' words:

I demand from you deeds of mercy which are to arise out of love for me. You are to show mercy to your neighbors always and everywhere.[5]

When a soul approaches me with trust, I fill it with such an abundance of graces that it cannot contain them within itself, but radiates them to others.[6]

---

4 *ibid.*, page 26

5 *ibid.*, page 25

6 *ibid.*, page 28

I now look at people differently. I am more attuned to the misery of others, and realize that I can often relieve their misery by showing love and compassion.

Since I have had this new understanding of God's mercy and made the message given to Faustina a part of me, my life has changed in many ways. I am aware that I can relieve the misery of others, putting God's love into action, even in simple ways like a phone call, a visit, a card. It may be just being aware of some pain or problems in the face of a checkout clerk at the grocery store. If I can smile and say a friendly word, perhaps it will make a difference. I see the needs in the lives of my friends, and I try not to be consumed by my well-being. My need and desire for God's mercy naturally flow into a desire to relieve the misery of others.

My prayer has changed. I pray for God's mercy (relieving my misery) for myself and family and others. It is like praying for Jesus to hug each of the people I am praying for and to give them exactly what they need in order to relieve whatever misery is plaguing them. It may be for my daughter who needs a job, or a friend with much pain due to cancer, or my brother-in-law with Parkinson's. Believing that Jesus knows just how to relieve their misery, I can trust Jesus with their care. Even when the prayers are not answered the way I think is best, I can trust that Jesus is in control and will take care of the people I love.

Whenever I get anxious about life events that I can't control, I force myself to let go and trust. This includes disagreements in my family, financial concerns, or CT scan results. This continual effort to trust and let go brings a sense of peace and a feeling of joy for living each day. I have an awareness of the good that has come to my life because of cancer. I don't feel alone anymore.

✺

Those who wait for the LORD shall renew their strength, they shall mount up with wings like eagles, they shall run and not be weary, they shall walk and not faint.

ISAIAH 40:31

✺

Dear Lord Jesus,
I know that you love me
—no matter what my sins.
I know that your mercy seeks to relieve
my misery—my cancer, my pain and hurts,
and I believe that when I call upon you
and trust in your great love for me
I can find true joy, peace, and happiness.
Please help me to extend this active love
to others, to heal, to comfort, to console,
to forgive, to remove pain.
Amen.

Dear Jesus,
I trust in you to be my strength for my journey.
Lord Jesus, have mercy on me.
Amen.

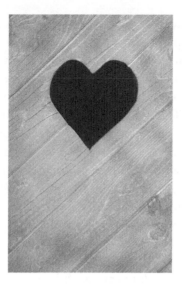

– Chapter Four –

What if...
Looking for Signs of an Afterlife

৵৯

Now if Christ is proclaimed as raised from the
dead, how can some of you say there is no resurrection of the dead? If there is no resurrection of
the dead, then Christ has not been raised; and if
Christ has not been raised, then our proclamation
has been in vain and your faith has been in vain.

1 CORINTHIANS 15:12–14

One day, while driving in the car, I was focusing on two people who had recently died. One friend talked about his faith in God and how he was ready to move on. He shared a little of his faith walk with me about a week before he passed away. He said, "Isn't this what we are all about? This life is just a steppingstone to what we are really meant for. I am looking forward to the joys of heaven. No pain. No cancer. I am really excited about meeting Jesus face to face." The other person faced his imminent death with trepidation. He continually stated that he wasn't yet ready. He did not want to die. He was afraid of what may or may not be lying ahead. He had no real belief in an afterlife. Just then, for a second, the thought crossed my mind, "What if my second friend was right?" I quickly recovered: I very much believe in an afterlife. A little later, I heard another friend, who was very religious all her life, voice the same "what if" question, and I realized that the desire for certainty about an afterlife can be a common need for those with serious illnesses.

In this chapter I share some contemporary signs that, for me, point to a world beyond this earthly life. They are signs seen in what our faith points to, as well as in present-day evidence of the supernatural.

For Christians, the primary, all-inclusive testimony to the existence of heaven and what awaits us is, of course, the Bible. Beginning with the story of creation, we hear about God's wonderful plan for us. The wonders of creation, nature, and human existence, are powerful signs that there must be a higher power in control of the universe. It is all too intricate and complicated to have just evolved by chance. Our daughter recently gave birth to our first grandchild. Thinking about the development of an embryo that began with one sperm and one ovum that is ultimately born into the world as a baby with a circulatory system, respiratory system, and everything else is truly miraculous. Our little granddaughter has not only a body, but a mind and spirit as well, and the soul dwells within the body.

The greatest feast of the Christian Church is Easter, when we celebrate Jesus' resurrection. The promise our faith gives us is that we also will share in the resurrection. Jesus promised his disciples, "And if I go and prepare a place for you, I will come again and will take you to myself, so that where I am, there you may be also" (John 14:3). There are many stories of resurrection appearances in the Scriptures. Could a group of believers spread the Christian faith so far and wide that it still exists 2,000 years later if it was merely a human construct? Most would agree that it is not only unlikely, but impossible. Our faith enables us to claim that Jesus opened wide the doors of heaven, and that we are welcomed there at the time of our death. "For we know that if the earthly tent we live in is destroyed, we have a building from God, a house not made with hands, eternal in the heavens" (2 Corinthians 5:1).

When I asked my high-school students how we know there is a heaven, at least one responded by pointing to apparitions of the Virgin Mary and other saints. The miraculous events that surround the appearances of the mother of Jesus cannot be rationally explained. People are healed in the waters of Lourdes. People flock to Fatima to be part of the events that have no earthly explanation. Reading and reflecting on the apparitions of the Blessed Mother can be reassuring and comforting, and reading about the lives of the saints can strengthen our faith.

Even though our faith gives us all we need in order to believe in an afterlife, some seek further signs. Just look at the fascination with the spirit world in our society today. Go into any bookstore and you will find book after book on appearances of angels, not to mention near-death experiences. In December 1993, *Time* turned its magazine cover over to angels, and featured an article that reported poll results of sixty-nine percent of Americans believing in the existence of angels. Angels have been the topic on *Oprah,* of TV news magazine shows and movies. One of the most popular shows right now is *Touched by an Angel.* People want to believe in angels. The concept of angels gives us hope and an assurance that we are not alone in this mixed-up world. Joan Wester Anderson has authored several collections of angel stories. When I really need a pick-me-up, I read a few of these stories. One of my favorite ones describes a young woman who was walking alone at night and was passing an evil-looking man. As she walked past him, she felt very afraid and foolish to be walking alone, because she had read news stories about a rapist in the area. The next morning she heard about a woman who had been attacked near the corner on which she saw the scary-looking man. She went to the police and helped to identify him in a lineup. Afterward, the officers asked the man why he didn't attack the first young woman. He replied that he would have been stupid to risk his life since she had two tall, strong men walking beside her.

Another popular topic for those searching for proof of an afterlife is near-death experiences (NDE). Dr. Raymond A. Moody pioneered research into the events that occurred in people who have been clinically dead and resuscitated or in people who have been very close to death. Moody writes of his research in his book, *Reflections on Life After Life* (Bantam, 1978). His investigation presents strong evidence of an afterlife. Many people report having a sensation of floating out of their body and being able to see and hear the events occurring around their body. All report having an incredible sense of peace and well-being. There is no pain, no awareness of any body sensation. Many report traveling through a dark tunnel to be met by a loving light that radiates total acceptance, compassion, and love. Some believe this light to be Jesus, and many experience a "life review" of understanding how their choices in life affected others. To many, it was a wonderful experience—a "glimpse of heaven"—and they did not want to return to this life. Many met relatives or friends who had died. They were told their mission was not complete, it was not their time, and they needed to return.

People tell of returning with a sense of peace and having no more fear of dying. They say they have a new sense of mission and a stronger sense of faith and of wanting God to be a real part of their lives. The experience is profound and life-changing.

Other signs of the existence of an afterlife are detailed in the book, *Final Gifts*, by two hospice nurses, Maggie Callanan and Patricia Kelley. After caring for many people with terminal illnesses, the authors report a common experience of their patients of being in the presence of someone not alive. Many patients know when death will occur, and some patients can control the timing of their death. Some people have out-of-body experiences as they near death. At the time my mother was nearing death, I walked into her room to sit with her. She was reaching into the air with her right hand. I asked her what she was doing, and she said her mom was just there. I thought, of course, she was hallucinating, and I told her that her mother had been dead for many years. That was before I read *Final Gifts*. My father had similar stories of his deceased brother visiting him to tell him it was time for him to follow. My dad replied that he wasn't going because he was "too yellow." And sure enough, Dad, at age eighty-eight, pulled out of his illness to live several more years.

I, too, have a story of Jesus' promise of resurrection. At ninety-five, my father was in a nursing home and in poor health for some time. One morning, my sisters and I were called to the home because my father stopped breathing for a short time, and they did not expect him to make it. After praying together throughout the day, my four sisters and I were sitting around our loving father's bed as it was getting close to midnight. We were tired, concerned, anxious for his passing over to the new life we believed was awaiting him. Suddenly, we all began to notice a strong fragrance that was only over our father's body. It was as if someone placed twelve dozen roses on his body. Each sister talked about the wonderful fragrance. We did not understand where it came from. No one had walked in the room. None of us had on perfume. And then, just as quick as it appeared, the fragrance disappeared with no lingering scent. It must have lasted only a few minutes. We wondered why we had been given this beautiful experience. One of my sisters then quietly told us that, only minutes before, she had asked God to show us a sign that there really was a heaven. We did receive a sign, and we believe we experienced a real miracle as we companioned our dad on his journey from this life to the next. We believe he is enjoying a better life in heaven with our mom with no pain or suffering—all that our faith promises us through the gift of Jesus' death and resurrection.

When I reflect on the threat of my own death from cancer, I read or listen to tapes of people's stories of near-death experiences. I put myself in the person's place and imagine myself being greeted by my guardian angel at death. I speculate on how it might feel floating above my body and letting my thoughts take me to the location of family members and then being escorted through the tunnel toward the amazing light. I envision Jesus meeting me at the end of the tunnel to give me a welcoming hug. We have a picture hanging in our hallway of Jesus in a white robe, surrounded by clouds and angels, reaching out with compassion and love to hug a person who recently died. That's exactly what I imagine happening to me. I often think about the beauty of heaven, the joy of seeing my parents again, and the experience of meeting two of our children—our daughter, Mary, who died shortly after birth, and a baby I miscarried early in the pregnancy. I marvel at the promise of indescribable beauty and joy, no fear, anxiety, or pain—and no cancer.

> If a tiny baby could think, it would be afraid of birth. To leave the only world it has known would seem a kind of death. But immediately

after birth, the child would find itself in loving arms, showered with affection and cared for at every moment. Surely the baby would say, "I was foolish to doubt God's plan for me. This is a beautiful life."

For the Christian, passing through death is really a birth into a new and better world. Those who are left behind should not grieve as if there were no hope. Life is changed, not taken away.

Our dear ones live on, in a world beautiful beyond anything we can imagine. With Jesus and Mary, they await the day when they will welcome us with joy.[7]

❦

Jesus said to her, "I am the resurrection and the life. Those who believe in me, even though they die, will live, and everyone who lives and believes in me will never die."

JOHN 11:25

What no eye has seen, nor ear heard, nor the human heart conceived, what God has prepared for those who love him.

1 CORINTHIANS 2:9

7 *A Word of Consolation,* The Marianist Mission Mount Saint John, 4435 East Patterson Road, Dayton, OH 45481-0001. Reprinted with permission.

Dear Jesus,
I wonder what heaven might be like.
I wonder what my friends and relatives
are experiencing in heaven. I am so grateful for
my faith. And I know I can believe your promise,
that I can look forward to sharing a new life with
you in heaven. Please let this belief bring me
comfort and peace as I struggle with my illness.
Welcome me with a loving hug when it's my time
to join you in heaven. Thank you for loving me.
Amen.

ℬ

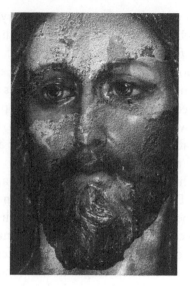

– Chapter Five –

Understanding God's Role in Our Suffering

❧

Jesus did not come to do away with suffering
or to remove it.
He came to fill it with his presence.

PAUL CLAUDEL (1868–1955)

In 1996, ten years since my previous surgery, my doctor called to tell me that I had a mass in my lungs and to schedule me for a biopsy. I cried, felt panic, fear, anger, why me?...not again! I considered myself a good person, a good mother, wife, sister, friend. I was involved in many volunteer activities that helped other people. Why would God, whom I considered a friend, do this to me? My initial reaction was to blame God. I felt abandoned. But was God really to blame?

I recall a high-school theology course I taught, called "Death and Dying." Students would often share how family members dealt with suffering in their lives. After teaching this course to more than 300 students, I realized that many people blame God for their suffering. If this view of God's role in suffering continues, their relationship with God is often destroyed, they lose their faith, and stop praying and going to church.

Rabbi Harold Kushner's best-selling book, *When Bad Things Happen to Good People*[8], uses Job's story of suffering to help us understand and clarify God's role in it. Kushner discusses the fallacies of seeing God as the one sending suffering to punish or to test our faith. If you haven't read this book, I urge you to do so. If you have, you might want to pick it up again.

I've heard it all. Some believe that God sends cancer or AIDS or Alzheimer's as a punishment for our sins. Then how do we explain the suffering of small children, those without sin? Jesus put this reasoning to an end

8 Harold S. Kushner, *When Bad Things Happen to Good People* (New York: Schocken, Avon, 1981).

when he was asked, "'Rabbi, who sinned, this man or his parents, that he was born blind?' Jesus answered, 'Neither this man nor his parents sinned; he was born blind so that God's works might be revealed in him'" (John 9:2–3). Then Jesus healed his blindness.

To question "why" is a common reaction to cancer or any other kind of suffering. But we can be assured that God does not send us cancer to punish us. Rabbi Kushner reinforces this belief by stating that we cannot believe in a God who is good and just and then believe that innocent people are inflicted with some sort of suffering as punishment. Therefore, if God is good, we cannot blame the victim or God for the punishment.

The same type of reasoning follows with regards to the fallacy that God sends suffering to test the victim's faith. Jesus, as the Son of God, shows us what God is like. Time and again, Jesus healed the crippled, the sick, the suffering, even curing the demonic. Jesus never inflicted pain or suffering, but went about healing out of love and compassion. He sometimes attributed the healing to the strength of faith (see Mark 5:25–34;10:46–52; Matthew 9:27–31;15:21–28; Luke 5:17–20;7:1–10). But Jesus never caused pain or suffering in order to test a person's faith. My faith was already strong when I was diagnosed with recurrence after recurrence. My relationship with God has changed, grown, and evolved into a deeper friendship through all the struggles and pain of fighting cancer. But this is a response to a situation, not the results of a test by God.

God never gives us more than we can handle. What a distressing way to see God and a terrible burden on survivors. Our baby daughter died shortly after birth, having only a partial brain and no back skull. If God only gives us what we can handle, then am I to blame for being strong enough to handle my child's death? If I were weaker would God have given me only healthy children? This view of God somehow places blame on the strong parent. A good and just God doesn't distribute pain and suffering—like cancer, AIDS, multiple sclerosis, or diabetes—as if dealing a deck of cards and giving the losing hand to those *who can take it.* Jesus even healed his enemies. We can believe that our God loves us and would never inflict pain or suffering because we can *handle it.*

Some believe that suffering happens so that we appreciate what we already possess. This does not describe the mindset of a compassionate, loving, giving, kind, generous God, a God who is likened to a loving parent who gives only good things to a child.

Kushner believes that bad things happen to people because of two primary forces: One is the free will of people; the other is the law of nature. These explain pain and suffering in the world. Much of our world's suffering is caused by the events triggered by human choices. Wars, famine, the Holocaust, poverty, crime are all caused by human beings, not God. When my friend's niece was killed by a drunk driver, it was not God who took this young sixteen-year-old's life. The man chose to drink and drive, and the result was the taking of an innocent life. When 100 people are killed in an airplane crash because of a terrorist bomb, the tragedy was caused not by God, but human choice. There does exist a tug between good and evil in our world. Often evil prevails and innocent people suffer.

When tornadoes flatten towns and hurricanes destroy homes, it is the result of the laws of nature. The meteorologists have explanations of how these events turn into natural disasters. There are over two hundred types of cancer, and research books on cancer explain multiple causes for each type. I have friends with mesothelioma. The primary cause of this cancer is asbestos. I believe that my cancer was triggered by stress, along with other unknown environmental or biological causes. Stress in my life lowered my immune system and my body was not able to destroy the cancer cells that were present. There are many diseases that are passed on by hereditary make-up. Nature, not God, is the contributing factor in sickness.

So, what is God's role in all the sickness and suffering in the world? God is not a passive bystander. God cries with us. God suffers along with us. God's role is to comfort, support, and console. Jesus walks with us on our journey, ready to help us carry our cross. We are human beings, created by God, living in this world governed by the laws of nature and shaped by the free will of human beings. God asks nothing of our existence to which his own son was not also exposed. Jesus endured ridicule and rejection, hate and contempt. Jesus endured being lonely, abandoned by his friends. He felt excruciating physical pain in his scourging and crucifixion. And Jesus, too, felt the abandonment of God and questioned why. "At three o'clock Jesus cried out with a loud voice, *'Eloi, Eloi, lema sabachthani?'* which means, 'My God, my God, why have you forsaken me?'" (Mark 15:34).

I am called, like Jesus, to put my faith and trust in God's hands. "Father, into your hands I commend my spirit" (Luke 23:46). When I feel most alone and fearful, I can place my cancer, pain, anguish, fear, into the loving, compassionate hands of God. In October of 1996, when I was facing my third recurrence in four months—and this time in my remaining kidney—I wrote in my journal:

Tonight I was so deeply touched. Eleven people
were here from church to pray with me. I couldn't
stop crying. What I felt was support, comfort,
and being wrapped in a blanket of love. I guess
my fears have been that somehow God wanted
me to die. What I realized tonight is that God
didn't cause my cancer and that God loves me.
Somehow I am called to carry my sufferings with
the same dignity as Jesus. I need to trust God
and believe that God is present through it all.

I believe God walks with me on my journey. I am called to "take up my cross" and follow in the footsteps of Jesus (see Luke 9:23). We each have a different burden to carry. Some have abusive marriages; some live in the prison of poverty; some have cancer or mental illness, Parkinson's, Alzheimer's, AIDS, and so on; others are alone in the world. Whatever our burden, we believe that God is our companion on this journey of life. We choose to believe what is promised us in Romans 8:28: "We know that all things work together for good for those who love God, who are called according to his purpose."

Early in my cancer journey, some well-meaning people questioned the strength of my faith. I was told that I would be healed of my cancer if my faith was strong enough—if I truly believed that God would cure me. After my second recurrence in 1986, a well-meaning Christian questioned my faith. She intimated that I was responsible for my own cancer spread because I must not have believed that God would cure me. I was hurt and offended by these comments.

God holds a deep love for each one of us and would never withhold healing because of our fears and uncertainties. In Matthew's Gospel, Jesus cured all who were ill. No mention is made of faith being the first requirement (see Matthew 8:16). I know many holy, faith-filled people who were not healed of their cancer.

Our faith calls us to ask for God's healing and then to trust that, whatever the outcome, God is with us. Somehow, out of our suffering comes the opportunity to bring good into the world. We are invited to model our suffering after Jesus. From the crucifixion came the resurrection. Jesus' death took on new meaning because of his resurrection. We, too, can bring new meaning to our cancer if we allow God to bring good out of it. Perhaps we are being given the opportunity to resolve hurting relationships, to stop taking a spouse for granted, or to take the time to show love and receive love in our lives.

My cancer recurrences have resulted in strengthening my marriage. Many nights I look over at my sleeping husband and realize this day is gone forever. Tomorrow will be another opportunity to embrace each moment and make the most of it. I want to spend time with him, just holding hands and watching TV. I value our time together, and my priorities have changed. If the house doesn't get cleaned, or dinner doesn't turn out right, I can shrug my shoulders and let go. My priorities are my family and friends, not in accomplishing or accumulating things.

Life is a mystery. Why do some people suffer and others seem to have it all? Why do some people receive a miraculous healing while others are allowed to die too young? Perhaps we die when our mission in this life is complete and it is our time to enjoy a new and wonderful life with God—an existence with no cancer, pain, or suffering. Sometimes we cannot make sense of it, nor can we explain it. I believe that God offers us the strength and peace we need to endure our suffering. God also offers us the peace and healing of our spirit, if not our physical bodies. "Then he said to them all, 'If any want to become my followers, let them deny themselves and take up their cross daily and follow me'" (Luke 9:23). Saint Paul's words of wisdom to the early Christians suffering persecution were: "I consider that the sufferings of this present time are not worth comparing with the glory about to be revealed to us" (Romans 8:18).

❧

Dear Jesus,
I know you also suffered much and that you call
me to follow you. Sometimes my suffering, fear,
and anxiety seem too much to bear. Please give
me the strength and the courage I need to fight
this cancer battle. Help me to turn my suffering
into good. Please comfort me and walk with me
on my journey.
Amen.

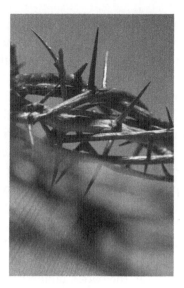

– Chapter Six –

Finding Value in Suffering

℘

Trust the past entirely to the mercy of God,
the present to his tender love,
and the future to his providence
and care over you.

AUGUSTINE OF HIPPO (354–430)

I recently returned from two weeks of cancer treatment in the Bahamas. This is one of the treatments that has helped me for two years. I made the trip alone for the first time. No one in my family could get away. Instead, I arranged to time my treatment with friends from Canada. They are like family—sharing the fight with cancer has created a strong bond between us. I let my friends choose from the two apartments we reserved. They chose the one with better air-conditioning, as I preferred fresh air. I was so disappointed when I walked into my apartment, because although there were many windows, only a few opened. I knew the apartment my friends were in not only had better air-conditioning, but also had windows that all opened and would provide a much better breeze. Then I noticed it. On the coffee table in my apartment was a large candle with the picture of the Blessed Virgin Mary (as shown on the Miraculous Medal in honor of the Immaculate Conception). And I knew that this was the apartment I was meant to have.

Although I brought several murder mysteries to read, I also brought a little booklet on the story of Fatima to reread. I wanted to have something for spiritual reflection during the trip. That candle was my constant reminder that I needed to read the booklet on Fatima, and not just have it take up space in my luggage. The second night, I began reading the children's story and found it hard to put down. This incredible story of Mary appearing to three shepherd children in Portugal in 1917 had meaning for my life today—in the year 2000.

Mary's message called the children to sacrifice much for the conversion of sinners and in reparation for sins against the Immaculate Heart of Mary and the Sacred Heart of Jesus. These children endured great suffering by giving up their lunches and water, by offering up their pain of being misunderstood, ridiculed, rejected, and even threatened. Lucia was ten years old, Francesco was nine, and Jacinta was only seven. The children's simplicity of belief really struck me. I had often thought I should not have to suffer because of my strong faith—after all, I have been faithful and loyal to God over the years. It's almost that I believed I deserved to be healed. And, if I were not healed of my cancer, then I should have an easy time of dealing with it, and an easy death. I didn't see my suffering as having any value.

The example of these little children showed me how wrong I was. Yes, God walks with me in my struggle with cancer, and God is my strength who brings me comfort and a sense of peace and joy. But I now see how I am called to take my sufferings and struggles and offer them up to God for the intentions of my family. I have always believed that my faith is my greatest gift. No one goes through life unscathed. Everyone has his or her own struggles and trials. It has always been my faith that has sustained me through it all. And I desire that same strength for my daughters and family. Therefore, I pray daily for a strong faith for my children and my family. My prayer is that my family will feel the love of Jesus deep within their hearts, believing that Jesus cares about every detail of their lives, and having such trust that they will allow Jesus to guide their choices in life. So my prayer is not just that my family will believe with their minds, but rather with their hearts. It's the heart kind of love that makes a difference in my life. Now I see that I can put some power behind those prayers. I can take my everyday struggles and pain with cancer and offer it all up to God for my family. My suffering has value!

Jesus offered up his passion and death as a sacrifice to God for the forgiveness of our sins and to open the doors to heaven. The sacrifice of his life destroyed the power of our bodily death and replaced it with the promise of new and eternal life. I began my new life in Christ in baptism, and at my earthly death I will be welcomed into the fullness of new life in Christ in my heavenly home. Jesus' suffering has meaning, and my suffering has meaning. The greatest love of all is to give up your life for others. What a love offering it is, then, to lift up my pain and struggles to God for the special intentions of my family.

The first two days in my beach-front apartment were very hot and with no breeze. I wasted time complaining to myself over having an apartment with so few windows that opened. Instead, I could have offered it up to God as a sacrifice for the deepening of my family's faith and for their special needs. Instead of feeling sorry for myself because I can no longer teach due to my illness, I could have offered this pain and sorrow up to God. I have become aware that my days are filled with things to offer up: my fatigue, my having to take up to twelve injections a day, and the pain of having the nurse stick me three times a day for my IV. Staying on my special diet and keeping to a detailed schedule for various treatments, often accompanied by discomfort, can be so distressing, annoying, tiresome, and just plain difficult. The story of Fatima helped me understand that there can be meaning to it all, a purpose beyond just grasping for my healing—one that touches the lives of the people I love the most.

The last page of the Fatima booklet puts my call to offer up my pain and struggles in perspective. "[People] need not perform heroic sacrifices as did the children of Fatima; rather, they must fulfill their daily duties in life. And because these duties are oftentimes hard and burdensome, they become works of penance and sacrifice." Jesus calls us to take up our daily cross and to follow in his steps. By carrying my crosses cheerfully and with the intent of offering them as a sacrifice to God, I am following Jesus.

One would think that these little children who were selected to hear the message of Fatima would be allowed to be free of pain and protected in their lives. But this was not to be the case. Francesco and Jacinta died just three years after the apparitions. Jacinta experienced a very long, painful illness, which she offered up to God. In Jacinta's words,

> I'm going to love Jesus a lot, and the Immaculate
> Heart of Mary, and pray for you [Lucia],
> for the Holy Father, my parents, brothers, sisters,
> for everyone who asked me, and for sinners.
> I love to suffer for the love of our Lord and our
> Lady. They love those who suffer for the conversion of sinners.[9]

℣℈

---

9 *The Story of Fatima* (Mother of Christ Crusade, Inc. Billings, Montana, 1947, Chapter XII [no page count]).

My pleas for healing were often rationalized with advice for God. I have often thought that my cancer has prevented me from teaching, and this has so saddened me that I thought what a waste this cancer has made of my life. I can no longer do something that I enjoyed and in which I was successful. I know I made a positive difference in the lives of my students. So I advised God that my healing would benefit many things besides my physical health. I could return to teaching and begin again to touch the hearts and minds of my students. However, after realizing that my suffering with cancer does have value, who's to say my prayers of sacrifice in having cancer are not doing a greater good than had I continued teaching? I would like to think I am irreplaceable as a teacher, but the truth is: I am not. My pastor recently gave a homily about looking at life's events from the perspective of eternity. Putting myself in the big picture of enjoying eternal life makes this life with cancer seem almost insignificant. I have the power to make a positive difference in this world, cancer or no cancer.

I recently watched an *Oprah* show that featured the story of a mother with cancer and the consequent effect on her children. After watching the show, I decided that I needed to apologize to our youngest daughter for "ruining" her teenage years. My surgeries and recurrences began again when she was just sixteen. She didn't have a "normal" mom for the last two years of high school. I was in treatment and even missed out on taking her to college and helping her set up her dorm room. My sister shopped with her to buy her necessities and to outfit her dorm room. To make it even worse, I missed taking her back the next fall also. In fact, I never even saw her living arrangements for her sophomore year in college. A few months ago, I took Debbie aside and apologized for taking away normal teenage time, and I apologized for her having a mom with cancer and the gloom that hung over her high-school and early-college years. She is twenty-one now and engaged. I thought I needed to give her permission to tell me off—or yell at my cancer—and put it behind her. I told her I would understand if she hated me for what I did to her, even if I did not hurt her intentionally. I guess I listened too closely to the TV psychologists, because Debbie responded that it was OK. She loved me, she didn't hate me for missing out on so much, and she didn't blame me for anything. In fact, she said, who knows whether having a mom with cancer had kept her from being a wild teen. It brought home the passage that "all things work together for good for those who love God" (Romans 8:28). The value of our suffering is not always easily detectable.

Many good things have occurred through my life with cancer. My relationships with my husband and children, sisters, and family are richer. I have made many good friends who also have cancer. Their examples of finding humor in our illnesses, maintaining positive attitudes, and persevering through pain and recurrences, have challenged and supported me. I am so grateful to know them and to share my journey with them. My faith has a simplicity and depth that I never imagined possible. Issues and problems are filtered through a lens that allows me to see clearly what is important and what is not. I cherish each day and am grateful for opportunities to make a difference in people's lives. I like the person I have become as a result of my cancer diagnosis. The dying and rising of Jesus—the paschal mystery—has meaning in my own life. Out of my suffering with cancer comes new life or good; out of the sacrifices I offer up in dealing with my illness comes potential for good.

The message of Fatima has taught me that my sufferings have value. This is certainly not what the world teaches. Our society tells us that suffering has no value and the sick are to be pitied. I may be healed, or I may not. Either way, my journey includes much pain and suffering, and I can offer it up to God for my family, friends, their needs, and faith relationship with Jesus. I feel as if I have wasted too much precious time complaining and feeling sorry for myself. I have talked about wanting to live and die with the same dignity as Jesus. Now I need to endure my suffering with the same dignity as Jesus, who loved us so much that he gave up his life for our sakes. I like this new perspective of sacrifice and suffering. It feels healthy and good.

꽃

Three times I appealed to the Lord about this, that it would leave me, but he said to me, "My grace is sufficient for you, for power is made perfect in weakness." So, I will boast all the more gladly of my weaknesses, so that the power of Christ may dwell in me. Therefore I am content with weaknesses, insults, hardships, persecutions, and calamities for the sake of Christ; for whenever I am weak, then I am strong.

2 CORINTHIANS 12:8–10

Dear Jesus,
It isn't easy to endure the pain and sufferings
that come with my illness. But, Jesus, your
example shows me that good can come out of my
suffering. Help me, O Lord, to unite my suffering
to yours. I offer up a willing sacrifice for a
deepening of faith for my friends and family.
Lead us all to experience your embrace
of love, forgiveness, and compassion.
Help me, O Lord, to find strength in my weakness,
and to allow your grace to be enough for me.
Amen.

☙

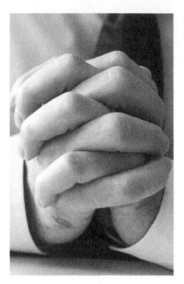

– Chapter Seven –

Connecting Through Prayer

ℬ

The value of persistent prayer is
not that God will hear us, but
that we will finally hear God.

WILLIAM J. MCGILL

Cancer helped me to stop taking God for granted and to begin putting my heart and soul into the relationship. When things were going well in my life, faith and trusting God came easy. The crisis of cancer turned my faith perspective inside out, and called me to deeper prayer experiences. The meaning of the sacraments came alive as did a new appreciation of various saints as potential intercessors and inspirations for accepting and living with my diagnosis. I began to listen to the word of God in the Scriptures not as stories of long ago, but as God's message to me now. Since my cancer diagnosis, the depth of my prayer has allowed God to touch the core of my innermost being. God and I are partners on this journey.

I remember trying to get across to my students that God was present to us in special ways in the sacraments, through grace. I wrapped a student up in a gold sheet and called her Grace. She had a sign pinned to her front that read "Grace," and a sign pinned to her back that read "God's Presence." I defined grace as God's loving presence, and used this live visual aid when I discussed the sacraments of baptism, confirmation, Eucharist, penance, anointing of the sick, marriage, and holy orders. I desperately wanted the students to understand that we are given a great gift in each of the sacraments— God's presence and love in a close and personal way. I remember teaching that the sacraments aid us in living our lives. When life gets tough, God is there to help us through the struggles.

Through my multiple cancer recurrences, my teaching has come back as a challenge and invitation to put my life where my mouth was then. My teachings about the sacraments are no longer mere words, but lived experience. Receiving a sacrament is a prayer experience of communicating my joys, sorrows, and needs to Jesus and, in turn, receiving the presence of Jesus that comforts, heals, forgives, and loves me. The touch, words, and presence of Jesus are all very real to me as I bring my trials to daily Mass; as I confess my sins in the sacrament of reconciliation, and ask for forgiveness and help to be a more loving person; and as I am anointed with oil to receive strength and healing for my body and soul.

When our granddaughter was recently baptized, I listened to the words of the deacon, and thought about the gift she was given that day—new life in Christ. I thought that no matter what happens in her life, she has Jesus walking beside her. She will never be alone. And I thought about the emptiness I would feel without Christ's presence in my life. The ups and downs of life are painful enough, but I endure them in the faith and belief that Jesus walks with me.

In addition to the sacraments being a source of strength and support, I have found that the lives of the saints and various relics have offered me comfort and inspiration. Upon hearing of my recurrences, many people sent cards that included prayers for healing and information about a saint, often accompanied by a medal or small fabric piece that touched the relic of the saint. Remembrances of Saint Ann, Father Solanus Casey, Mother Mary Clelia, Saint Peregrine, Saint Thérèse of the Little Flower, and Saint Philomena are reminders of the faith and love of others. I would ask and pray for the intercession of these saints before my surgeries, and I would tuck a scapular in my socks and let the nurses know that I wanted it with me at all times. I received much consolation in believing that Mary and the saints were watching over me as the doctors operated.

When my doctor first suspected a return of my cancer in 1996, my pastor lent me a small three-dimensional antique silver cross that is said to contain a piece of wood that touched a relic of the true cross. This little cross brought me hope, and I clutched it in my hand each night as I went to sleep. It made me think of Jesus' pain and suffering and that I was not alone. Jesus knew my fears and would help me face whatever the future held. The little silver cross was inviting me to unite my pain and suffering with his. I think that reminder of the cross helped me endure the endless waiting for phone calls, decisions and information from a variety of doctors, the biopsies, brain scans, bone scans, and three surgeries within five months. When I couldn't pray because I was too frozen with fear, I could still hold that small cross and somehow feel connected to Jesus.

On one of my many trips to the health food store, I began talking with a lovely elderly lady, named Margaret, who serviced the vitamin and supplement section. She shared a little of her husband's story with me. He had prostate cancer and was trying many natural things, but they were very afraid he was getting worse. She reached into her pocket and unfolded a scrap of paper. On it was written "Ps. 118:17." She said another customer had told her to place copies of this Scripture quote in various places around the house as encouragement. This customer saw this practice as combining the art of positive thinking with the power of God's word. I scribbled the Scripture notation on my receipt. As soon as I got home, I grabbed my Bible, wondering what the message would be. "I shall not die, but I shall live, and recount the deeds of the Lord." I repeated it over and over again. I told my sister, and she laminated little signs with the passage for me to place all over our house. I have it on my dresser mirror, on the refrigerator, in the family room, near the computer, and so on. Each time I pass the sign I silently pray the passage, "I, Jeanne, shall not die, but live to praise the Lord."

Other Scripture passages often hit me as being just for me at the time. It's like I am listening to God speak to my heart. When I was diagnosed with my inoperable tumors in May 1998, I was so caught up in fear that I couldn't pray. I needed others to keep praying for me, but I was very afraid people would give up on me. I thought people would think the writing on the wall was such that I was not going to make it, and then they would stop praying for me. Acquaintances would stop me in the grocery store or drugstore, and say how sorry they were for me. I always responded by asking them to keep praying for me. I asked my students not to give up on me, but to keep praying. Gradually, people from my parish and friends and family assured me that they were not giving up, but storming heaven with many prayers. The Gospel reading at Mass that week was from Mark's Gospel about the paralyzed man being lowered through the roof by friends in order for Jesus to heal him. "When Jesus saw their faith, he said to the paralytic, 'Son, your sins are forgiven...I say to you, stand up, take your mat and go to your home'" (Mark 2:5,11). When the paralyzed man could not go to Jesus alone, his friends carried him there. When I was so fearful and worried about yet more tumors, I was unable to go to Jesus alone. My friends carried me there with their prayers. Believing people had faith that Jesus could heal me stilled my mind and allowed me to rest in the assurance that I was being brought to Jesus in prayer.

I strongly believe in the power of prayer. I want to relate two stories from my own life that verify that truth for me. In 1986, I was two years past my original kidney surgery for cancer. I felt good, and the doctors assured me that they had "gotten it all." However, I had this intuition that something was not quite right. I started praying and asking God to help me find out what, if anything, was wrong. I went to my gynecologist for an exam, and she said she thought one of my ovaries was different. She took an ultrasound, which resulted in her recommending surgery to remove an abnormality in my ovary. The second opinion doctor told me I had a perfectly formed ovary, and he did not recommend surgery. His ultrasound showed no abnormality. It came down to my call. I prayed very hard about it, and then decided to have the surgery.

My family and friends all banded together to pray during the surgery. On opening me up, the surgeon was stunned to see a perfectly formed ovary. She almost closed me up, then and there, but something nagged at her to take out the ovary anyway and send it to be checked. Before she finished closing up, the pathology report came back: kidney cancer—a metastasis from two years ago! She immediately performed a full hysterectomy. After the surgery, she couldn't explain the decision to remove the ovary and have it checked. I see God's hand in guiding the surgeon to make good decisions.

Ten years later, the CT scans indicated tumors in both lungs. What a panic! Until that time, all my tumors were easily removable. How in the world could I lose my lungs? It wasn't like losing an ovary or one of my kidneys. Prayers started, and I was on every prayer list imaginable in St. Louis and even in other parishes around the country. My sisters had a lot of contacts! The doctor scheduled me for a biopsy since it had been ten years since my last cancer surgery. They thought it was unlikely that I had a recurrence of kidney cancer. I came out of the biopsy with one lung a little collapsed due to the procedure, but hearing the report from the doctor that there was no tumor in the other lung. The doctors couldn't explain it, and supposed that the original CT scan had picked up a rib by mistake. Thank you, God.

I was now a good candidate for surgery, with the risk that I could lose one lung. Prayers continued nonstop. After surgery, I could not believe the report. The tumor was not in my lung (even though I had the biopsy and CT scans that showed it was). Rather, the tumor was behind my lung, leaning on a lymph node and was easily removed. So, here I was, in lots of pain, but happier than I ever thought possible after cancer surgery. I still had both lungs and everything had gone well. I may not have been miraculously healed of my cancer, but I certainly felt the presence and power of prayer and the healing power of God.

My sense of God's presence in my life is very real. I am aware of it in the little things of each day and in the big events. I try to walk daily while praying the rosary and the Chaplet of Divine Mercy described by St. Faustina Kowalska. In attending daily Mass, I lay my concerns and petitions at the foot of the altar when I enter church. I often write in my journal to assist me in identifying feelings. Looking back over various entries helps me see how I have grown, and to understand how God has been present in my life. It is second nature to me now to talk to God when driving or cooking. I try not to make decisions without asking for God's help. I have a process that I use to make decisions with God's help. It includes:

- Inviting God to be a part of the situation and help me make the right decision
- Gathering all the facts and listing the pros and cons
- Seeking advice from people I respect and who may be knowledgeable in the area
- Reflecting on what my heart says
- Making a decision and letting it sit for a day to see if I feel at peace

Inviting God's presence and participation in the decision-making process gives me the assurance that I'll know, deep in my heart, what is right or wrong for me. This process applies in my life, whether I'm deciding on surgery, a treatment option, or even buying a car.

Centering prayer, or prayer of contemplation, allows me simply to sit silently in the presence of God. The result is the gift of peace from Jesus. When I feel disturbed by my situation, I close the door to our bedroom and take thirty minutes without thinking—just to spend time with Jesus. In centering prayer, I still my mind and body to acknowledge the presence of God within me. There are no words to memorize or formulas to learn. Without trying to do anything, the person who centers takes on God's peace and joy for living each day. I combine my time for centering prayer with my healing meditations. After quieting my body through the relaxation technique, and inviting Jesus into my body for healing my cancer through visualization, I then sit quietly in prayer. Sometimes I use a mantra, often only the word, "Jesus." Any thoughts that come to me are just allowed to exit my mind. I do not dwell on any topics or thoughts, but use the mantra to focus on quiet prayer. I am aware of Jesus' presence within me, and the time is spent simply sitting silently with him. It is deep, personal prayer with God. I come to God as I am and allow God to be a part of me. This quiet time with God helps me know the peace that I long for in the face of my cancer. God touches me in a very personal way, to heal my spirit.

ॐ

Prayer is exhaling the spirit of man and
inhaling the spirit of God.

EDWIN KEITH

ॐ

Dear Lord,
I want you to partake more in my life.
I need to believe and know with my heart
that you are with me. Help me to listen and hear
you speak to me. Send me your Spirit that I may
come to know you in a more personal way.
Teach me to make my life a prayer.
Amen.

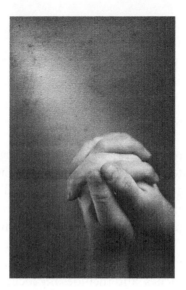

– Chapter Eight –

The Healing Hand of God

❧

WHAT CANCER CANNOT DO

Cancer is so limited—
It cannot cripple love
It cannot shatter hope
It cannot corrode faith
It cannot destroy peace
It cannot kill friendship
It cannot suppress memories
It cannot silence courage

It cannot invade the soul
It cannot steal eternal life
It cannot conquer the spirit.

AUTHOR UNKNOWN

৯১

Many medical experts (Dr. Bernie Siegel, Dr. Carl Simonton, Dr. Joan Borysenko, to name a few) write about the power of meditation to facilitate healing of cancer tumors. After reading many excellent books on meditation and cancer, using several different audio tapes, and attending relaxation/visualization workshops, I designed my own healing visualization that combines various approaches, and includes my focus and need to have God participate and direct my healing.

I imagine myself sitting in the center of my head, checking control panels of my immune system for cancer, to see that all levers are up, and checking my immune system for colds, and so on, and that all those levers are up. Jesus is present in the image of the Sacred Heart. He joins me, faces me, and we touch hands. I feel energy and power transferred to me. Jesus is my guide.

Sometimes he talks to me and we join hands and travel down my neck and chest to inspect my thymus gland (the center of my immune system), kidney, lungs, and so on.

First we arrive at the thymus gland. It is guarded and cared for by an angel that I've named Uriel. Uriel shows us how the white blood cells are killing cancer cells. As the white blood cells enter the thymus gland, they exit as gold angel warriors. Uriel turns off the light in my body so that I can see how effective and numerous my angel warriors are. Usually my whole body is gold. I thank Uriel, and Jesus and I go on to my kidney.

My kidney is guarded by another angel, Michael. Sometimes we join hands and watch the gold angels that cover the kidney. They are trying to heal the scar tissue, but aren't sure how. They are using vitamin E to coat the kidney to get rid of the scar tissue. Then I see the warrior angels attack the cancer cells in the kidney, brain, lungs, and lymph nodes with their swords. When they do this, the cancer cells turn a listless gray—empty and dead.

I then imagine the dead cancer cells being washed out of my body through my bladder and urinary tract. There's a drain for the cancer cells coming out of the bladder.

I picture me in the present, healthy and cancer-free. I'm smiling and sometimes dancing. Finally, I visualize myself in the future, usually as a grandmother enjoying my family and grandchildren. After that, I just sit quietly, silently, in the presence of Jesus.

Sometimes different images come to me that address specific needs. One day I was feeling particularly sorry for myself having cancer (I call this my private pity party). In my meditation, Jesus entered my body, ushering in thirty or forty hearts. These hearts, Jesus told me, represented the love and prayers of all my friends in heaven. This was to remind me that I was not alone, many people cared for me, and many people in heaven were praying and pulling for me.

Another meditation that I frequently use is to imagine a large heart entering my body from the top of my head. This heart represents all the love, prayers, and concern present in the people I know on earth—all my students, friends, family, people from my church, and neighbors. This love is more powerful than any cancer, and the heart goes through my body upside-down. As the heart nears a cancer cell, the heart opens at the rounded "V" and devours the cancer cells. This powerful heart of love travels throughout my body, claiming all cancer cells along the way. Then the large heart exits through the top of my head and takes away all the cancer cells.

At times I listen to Jesus give me a message of hope or comfort before we begin traveling through my body. I frequently receive a hug from Jesus. It seems so real that I've even had tears flow from my eyes. I encourage you to experiment with my meditations, and to create your own. It might feel strange at first, but in time you will receive consolation and hope.

ঌ

GUIDELINES FOR A HEALING MEDITATION

1. Choose a quiet place (perhaps play soothing instrumental music). Sit in a chair, back straight, with feet flat on the floor, arms resting on your lap. Close your eyes. Take four deep, cleansing breaths by inhaling and filling your lungs and abdomen. As you exhale, feel the air exiting your stomach and leaving your lungs.

Be aware of any tenseness in your forehead and facial muscles. Tighten the muscles and then let them relax. Continue doing this, and work your way down to your toes, tightening muscles and relaxing them.

2. Picture a warm liquid color entering the top of your head and moving down to fill your body. As it fills your body, be aware of how relaxed and peaceful you are.

3. Imagine yourself so small that you fit inside the center of your head. You are sitting in a relaxed, open posture. Let your imagination take over as you meet Jesus inside your head. Be aware of what Jesus looks like, his facial expression, the warmth in his eyes, and so on. Invite Jesus to travel through your body to heal the cancer cells. Take as long as you need.

4. Picture the cancer cells draining out through your bladder.

5. Picture yourself healed and well in the present.

6. Picture yourself healed and well in the future.

7. Conclude with simply resting in the presence of Jesus, with no thoughts, words, or images. You may wish to begin this part with saying "Jesus" in sync with your breathing. Rest in God's presence for five to twenty minutes.

֍

Be still, and know that I am God.

PSALM 46:10

Dear Lord Jesus,
I want you to be a part of my healing.
Please help me to welcome your presence in
my body to strengthen me and to conquer the
cancer cells. Give me the time and the quiet to sit
silently in your presence to visualize your help in
eliminating the cancer. Jesus, you never failed to
heal anyone who came to you, and I ask for your
healing hand to bring me wellness.
Amen.

ॐ

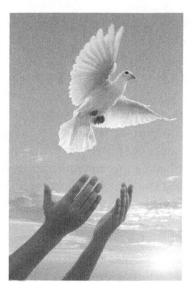

– Chapter Nine –

God Reaches Out

ఖ

When one door (of happiness) closes,
another one opens, but we look so long at
the closed door that we do not see the one
which has been opened for us.

HELEN KELLER (1880–1968)

I am a control person. For a control person to deal with cancer can be most difficult, because of the sense of helplessness regarding the ultimate outcome as well as with many areas along the way. I wish for instant answers, a miraculous cure, money to appear as needed, and so on. In asking God to reach out to me, it took a while to realize that God was indeed touching my sorrowful soul, my fearful spirit, my breaking heart, by sending love and concern and support from people around me. God was reaching out to me, perhaps not by appearing before me, but through the tangible touch of others.

Initially after my three surgeries in 1996, I thought I had it all together because of my supportive family and friends and my active faith. I visited a cancer-support center, the Wellness Community, for tai chi classes. Before beginning the session, the instructor asked each participant to go around the room and introduce him or herself with name and type of cancer. When it was my turn, I could not get it out. I was supposed to say, "Jeanne Martin, kidney cancer." I just cried instead. Rather than feeling foolish, I felt understood. That night I called to ask for a place in a weekly support group. My tears told me I had a lot of issues to work through.

I stayed in the group for thirteen months, and the weekly meetings became very important to me. I found that I wanted to say things that I couldn't say even to my husband. This group of people with cancer really understood the issues I encountered in my disease. They also challenged me. And they allowed me to be "me"— looking death in the face, and rethinking what life's all about. This is what I wrote in my journal at the end of the thirteen months:

This group taught me a lot, helped me cope with my fears, my feelings, my tears. I've learned that I need to live for more reasons than for my children. My life has value beyond being a mother. I've learned to let go of what doesn't really matter in life—like soda on the carpet, wrinkles around my eyes, old worn kitchen floor, a week of rainy weather, students who don't pay attention.

I've learned to greet the ordinary and appreciate the gift and joy of living...like having kids who spill drinks in the family room, being grateful for another day, month, year of living on this earth; for my age and the wisdom that comes with it. I'm grateful for the rain, the clouds, whatever the weather. I'm grateful just to live. Now, when my students aren't paying attention, I wonder what's bothering them...their struggles, fears, concerns that occupy their minds. I know what it's like to have your mind wander and to not be able to focus your attention on anything.

My support group taught me that my feelings of being helpless and being panicked at not having control in my life are normal. We became family, sharing each other's struggles, challenging each other, and supporting one another on our common journey.

God continued to reach out to me through my high-school students and fellow teachers. I was expecting kidney surgery in November 1996 with a six-week recovery. Our school happened to have an all-student assembly a few days after my diagnosis. I spoke to our entire student body of five hundred teenage girls, acknowledging my cancer and asking for their prayers and support. This was one of the most difficult and humbling experiences of my life. Here I was, their teacher, the one who was supposed to have all the answers, now having no answers. The one who seemed so strong was now broken and weak. I cried, and they cried. I taught two more weeks while I waited for surgery. I was overwhelmed by their cards, notes, prayers, and hugs. I can now see that they were touched by my openness and willingness to ask for help and prayers. That life lesson was more important than any lesson I carefully prepared for my classes.

God was not only reaching out to me, but turning my cancer diagnosis into an opportunity to reach out to others. I learned some of my students had parents with cancer. My openness encouraged these young, hurting girls to share their fears and their pain. When I was diagnosed with my recurrence in May 1998, the members of the senior class each wrote me a note and had them bound together. I treasure those loving messages. The support I received from the students and faculty gave me the encouragement not to give up.

It was difficult being open about my diagnosis. At times I felt as though I had a big scarlet C burned into my forehead and back. I imagined people were whispering and pointing at me. Then the cards, dinners, and supportive phone calls came in. People cared. People cared about me. I wasn't alone. Friends and acquaintances put me in contact with other cancer patients who beat the odds. I started hearing about hopeful cures. All I wanted were prayers, and I received that plus potential treatment options and unlimited love.

God's unconditional love and support are very apparent to me through the untiring efforts of my four sisters. Not only did they encourage me to fight and not give up, but they spent hours and hours researching treatments and gathering information. They listened to my fears and joined their tears with mine. My sisters showed me how to find God's strength and courage. They prayed with me and for me, and accompanied me to healing services. They gave up a week to be my companion for my ten weeks of alternative treatment. My sisters are such unselfish, generous friends that they made money from my dad available for my initial treatment. And after our dad died, they insisted on an even distribution of the assets, thus giving me the original funds as a gift. My sisters, Mary, Rosie, Betty, and Linda, are truly God's gifts to me. One of the greatest gifts of my illness has been recognizing my need for other people and accepting their love and support. My friends are organizing fund-raisers to help with our exorbitant medical expenses. I was reluctant to accept their generous offer of support, because my pride told me that I should be self-sufficient and independent, not needy or a charity case. The old adage of it being easier to give than to receive was certainly true in my situation of accepting the gift from these fund-raisers. Not only do I have the best sisters in the world, I also have the best friends. I am truly overwhelmed by the love, kindness, and generosity of others. The students from my high school participated in some fund-raisers to ease my financial burden. In a very real sense, I am experiencing the love of Jesus through the reaching out of others. The benefits of being open have definitely outweighed the detriments, for example, inappropriate questions, comments, feeling embarrassed, or pitied. Knowing that people cared sparked the inner courage I needed to fight for my life.

❧

When you say a situation or person is hopeless, you are slamming the door in the face of God.

CHARLES L. ALLEN

❧

Dear Lord,
Thank you for reaching out to me through
other people. When they love me as I am and
listen to my cries, I know you are there.
Sometimes it is so hard to be on the
receiving end. I'd much rather be the one giving.
Please help me to be open and to accept
the love and support of my family and friends.
And help me to enrich their lives by my example.
Amen.

❧

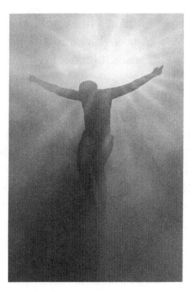

– Chapter Ten –

Feeling as if Time Is Running Out...
Peace Is My Gift to You

৵৶

Peace I leave with you;
my peace I give to you.
I do not give to you as the world gives.
Do not let your hearts be troubled, and do
not let them be afraid.

JOHN 14:27

Cancer turns a person's life upside down, at times robbing you of your life, and—without doubt—robbing you of your tranquility. Since being diagnosed with cancer in 1984, resulting in seven subsequent diagnoses of new tumors or growth, my topsy-turvy life is no longer marked by birthdays, anniversaries, holidays, or special events like family marriages; rather, the days, weeks, and months are set apart by my scheduled CT scans and MRIs. The dreaded anticipation is almost worse than facing an unfavorable outcome. I live between cancer tests. My life is sectioned off in three-, five-, or six-month segments. I feel the most relaxed when I have no test scheduled, as I can then almost pretend I'm normal or healthy, even if only for a short time.

But I can't pretend for long. I was never so aware of the lack of peace in my life as when I was diagnosed with cancer, and at the first four recurrences. My body showed the signs of anxiety and fear, both in anticipation of the tests and in facing the grim news. I would get heart palpitations. My breathing was labored, and at times I felt as if I could not get enough air. There was a tightness in my chest and lungs. Before surgeries, I often had "butterflies" racing through my stomach at the very thought of the operation. I longed for a feeling of peace. I was so caught up in the "what if" scenarios that I just could not relax. Peace—something so simple, yet so unattainable when we yearn for it desperately.

My seventh diagnosis of new tumors, in June of 2000, was the first time that I experienced peace while facing a dismal future. From the very center of my heart I felt calm, peaceful, and ready to let God lead me to finding treatment. What a contrast to my previous responses of anguish, hysterical crying, and fear! It did not take long to find out that I need an ongoing, trusting relationship with God to keep that peace in my heart. Peace is not just something I find once, but rather a gift I unwrap in the circumstances of each new day, especially those days marked by my cancer tests and visits to the doctor.

When these most recent scans showed four new tumors—yet another in my kidney, three around my pancreas, and growth in my chest tumor—I underwent very aggressive and expensive alternative cancer treatments for several months. My new doctor was very optimistic, and I felt intensely hopeful. Deep within, I told myself that if these treatments did not work, I probably had no other options. At the time, I saw these treatments as a "last chance" therapy. So when I scheduled my scans to measure the status of my cancer in November 2000, I told no one. I took the tests in secret. I had never done this before. I wanted to set my own time frame for telling friends and family of any poor results. I now know that was a mistake. Sitting in the hospital radiology waiting room was such a lonely experience. No one knew I was there, not even my husband. And no one knew to pray for me that morning. I wished I had the comfort and support of the prayers and thoughts of my family and friends. There was something missing that day.

Even though I told Jesus I trusted him with my life and the timing of my death, and I felt peaceful resting in the knowledge that Jesus was in control, I still felt anxiety facing the tests and hearing the results. I found I had to pray almost constantly to maintain my sense of calm or peace at my core and to keep the foreboding thoughts away.

My hopes and expectations for a decrease in my tumors were futile. When I heard the results, I felt as if I'd been punched in the stomach. It's not that I had major growth. I didn't. But I did not have any improvement—and I had told myself this was my last chance! To make matters worse, this radiologist counted the tumors in my kidney and wrote that in the report. Eight tumors in my kidney was the estimate! Multiple sounded so much "better" in previous reports. Eight seemed too exact, too many. How much longer could my kidney function normally? Now I felt as if time was running out.

Where did the peace go? It did not make sense to have peace and at the same time feel so weak, lacking control of my cancer, and so sorrowful at the prospect of leaving my family. I felt such confusion inside of me. I had to ask myself whether I still believed Jesus loved me, listened to, and answered my prayers? Whether I truly believed that Jesus walked with me, and that nothing could happen to me that Jesus did not allow? And whether, finally, I truthfully trusted Jesus with my life and the outcome of my treatments? Yes, I truly did believe all this, but I still felt an incredible sadness, weakness, and powerlessness.

I went to church early every day the week after I got my results. I went early enough to sit in the presence of the Blessed Sacrament between 7 and 8 a.m. I pretty much just sat there, sifting through my questions, and searching for some understanding of having what I thought were conflicting emotions of peace, trust, sadness, weakness. On the third day of just sitting in church and staring at the host contained in the ornate monstrance, I realized I also felt hurt. I had expected Jesus to be behind my cancer treatments that would, without doubt, provide a successful outcome, leaving me healed to live a long life. It was such a blow to feel as if time was running out because my friend, Jesus, didn't come through as expected. Even though I said I trusted Jesus, and I felt peaceful that Jesus was walking with me, I had also held certain requirements of what was best for my life and my family. I realized how unfair it was for me to say I trusted no matter what, yet down deep hold specific expectations.

Sitting in church examining my feelings that day, I imagined that it wasn't a host I was staring at, but a person. In my imagination, Jesus walked down the aisle of church, came into my pew, sat beside me, and took my hand. Then I knew it was OK again. I could feel sad and weak, yet strong and comforted in knowing Jesus was with me. I could feel the peace of Jesus' presence in my life, partnering me through my cancer experience, giving me permission to feel disappointment and hurt in the outcome, while still trusting Jesus to lead and guide me along the way. It reminded me of the poem, "The Tandem Bike Ride" (see Appendix B). Allowing Jesus to take the front seat of the tandem bicycle, he leads the way by comforting and encouraging me along the way in all the events of my life. No matter where I am on this crazy ride, Jesus is with me. I won't crash, and he never abandons me even when the ride will come to an end.

Forgiveness is a topic emphasized by almost every expert dealing with healing and wellness. The mind/body/spirit authorities discuss the importance of forgiveness in all areas of our lives in order to provide an atmosphere of peace, which is a prerequisite for healing. I recently heard a physician's report on television that outlined important choices for cancer patients. In addition to diet specifics, he first talked about the detrimental effects of such feelings as bitterness, guilt, anger, resentment, and blame. Forgiveness was recommended as the most important step to take in battling cancer. Last summer, we celebrated Mass in my home to pray for my healing. The priest stressed the importance to all who attended, as well as myself, to first focus on forgiveness before we come to God to ask for healing. We were asked to reflect on our sins, and ask God for forgiveness. In addition, we were asked to think about our lives and any person we needed to forgive or ask for forgiveness. When I thought about it later, it made sense that if I were bold enough to ask God for something so important as sparing my life, then I should first be willing to strive to set my relations right in the eyes of God. How could I ask God to heal me if I was not interested in healing my relationships?

By temperament, I have a rather smug attitude toward forgiveness. As a young person, I often held grudges, judged others, and withheld my forgiveness until the other person got the point and apologized. Over the past thirty years, I have steadfastly worked on being a more open, kind, less judgmental, and a more forgiving person. So whenever the topic of forgiveness is brought up, I usually think, "been there, done that." But when I was diagnosed with my recurrences in 1996, I began to reexamine my attitudes toward forgiveness.

This time my focus was around my cancer circumstances. Did I, on some level, blame myself or others for my cancer illness? My inability to handle stress? The stresses in my life? Did I hold some bitterness toward God for my situation?

During this particular Mass, I knew I was being asked to go deeper and reflect on any areas of forgiveness that needed attention in my life. I've learned to never think, "been there, done that" again. I have learned to value the sacrament of reconciliation as an aid to reflect on my life, let go of my mistakes and sins, and to ask for God's grace to live a life of love. This sacrament helps me maintain a feeling of peace in my life. After reflecting and confessing my sins, I feel a burden is lifted, and the presence of God touches me in a very personal way to help heal my spirit, and peace is the special outcome.

In facing cancer, I naturally see life through a different lens. Issues that may otherwise have been important, now seem insignificant. Life is too short to make the issue more important than the relationship. My cancer helps me to put events in perspective. I cannot rest thinking I've hurt another, even accidentally, and I find that I am much more willing to let go of events that may cause me hurt and to not condemn or judge others for the situation. I not only concur with the wellness experts—I believe that Jesus calls me to forgiveness in the big and little things of life. Only when my relationships are healthy, can I focus on healing my body. The burden of carrying hurts prevents me from attaining peace, and from being truly free to face my illness and focus on my treatment and healing.

Forgiveness can even work miracles. Peter Shockey tells an incredible story of the power of forgiveness in *Reflections of Heaven*. A man's twenty-three-year-old son was comatose from severe head trauma and brain damage after having been brutally attacked. The father was filled with rage and anger, and was determined to find the attackers to take revenge. He went to church, on the Sunday morning following the attack, consumed with hate and vengeance. The father caught a couple of words in the sermon that seemed to hit him directly. The sermon was on forgiveness. Realizing he couldn't go to God to ask for healing without first forgiving the men who beat his son, he prayed for God to help him forgive. He was so overcome by the message that he wept. The father went directly to visit his son after the church service, and was shocked to see him awake and healed of much of the head trauma. The doctors had no medical explanation for the turnaround. Forgiveness is powerful, life-changing, and healing—both spiritually and physically. God supplies the grace we need to let go of our hurt and anger.

A woman I know was diagnosed with cancer after she had been through a very difficult divorce. She told me she held on to the hurts that her husband's words had inflicted by replaying them daily in her mind. She felt worthless. Her financial future seemed hopeless, and she felt she had no control over the divorce settlement. After her diagnosis of cancer, she realized the importance of putting the past behind her and letting go of the pain. She made a decision to forgive him and move on to focus on her treatment.

To forgive and not to judge others are not easy tasks. God's grace helps me to forgive and to see others with eyes of compassion. Prayer enables me to reach out to God and ask for the strength and courage to forgive and to put aside my own pride in asking for forgiveness. Jesus is my model of forgiveness. He never justified withholding his forgiveness, even to those who betrayed and murdered him. My prayer each day is to be a channel of God's love in the world, and to put on the mind and heart of Jesus—the wisdom and courage to make right choices.

I ask to receive the sacrament of the anointing of the sick periodically. This sacrament is meant to strengthen and heal both physically and mentally. My family and I also attend healing services that usually include this healing sacrament. The priest lays hands on my head and prays for a healing of my cancer. Sometimes I am so touched that I cry throughout the service. I am aware of the presence and healing power of God in the praise and prayer of those in attendance. I leave with a deep feeling of God's presence and peace, knowing and believing that God is in charge of my life. I no longer need to focus on feeling helpless, because God is present in my illness, and I do not walk this journey alone.

Not long ago, I heard a simple song on a Christian radio station. There were just three lines to the song: "I believe, I adore, I trust." How simple that message is. And those three phrases seem to wrap up my faith journey with cancer. I believe that Jesus is God-with-us. As such, Jesus enters into my suffering with cancer by his suffering on the cross. I can most assuredly adore or praise this wonderful God who loves me so much. And I trust that God never leaves me alone. He never abandons me. I trust in God to make sense out of something that makes no sense to me, and to care for my family when I am no longer here. I trust Jesus to allow my life to have value in spite of—or because of —my cancer. Ultimately, I trust that God's plan is superior to mine (although I plan to have a long talk with him one day). I have found that when I try to take back control of my life's events and diminish the trust, I lose my peacefulness. It helps me to whisper this simple refrain whenever my peace seems shaky or my day is rocky. Lately, I have prayed these phrases when I heard about a cancer friend's bad report or listened to a TV newscast about cancer death statistics. "Jesus, I believe, I adore, and I trust in you." Peace, gentle, calming, freeing peace. What a gift of my faith in Jesus!

The Gospel of Luke tells a story of a woman who was sick for eighteen years (Luke 13:10–17). She is described as being "bent over and was quite unable to stand up straight" (verse 11). Perhaps she had severe osteoporosis with dowager's hump, making her back and shoulders so curved that she was forced to walk bent over; or maybe she had damage to the vertebrae in her back that caused the disability. Whatever it was, the disability prevented the woman from standing upright and seeing life clearly, meeting life head-on. The crippling illness would not allow the woman to interact with life as a normal person. This story can provide a reflection for us to symbolically name what is happening in our lives. Is my cancer causing me to be "bent over," preventing me from seeing life clearly, and interacting with others? If so, what do I need in order to stand upright?

As seen in these pages, I have found that some important answers to these questions may be found in

- My belief in a loving God and a closer relationship with God
- My trust in a God who wants to relieve my misery
- The support and prayers of friends and family
- My interaction with other people with cancer
- My accepting forgiveness from God and/or others
- My letting go of past hurts or blame

We are invited to bring all of our infirmities to God and place them in the divine care, thus receiving the peace that is beyond all understanding.

ॐ

"Thus says the LORD who made you, who formed you in the womb and will help you: Do not fear."

(ISAIAH 44:1–2).

Dear Jesus,
I very much want to feel your peace in my life.
Please reveal to me those areas that I need to
attend to. Lead me to full forgiveness and recon-
ciliation in all my relationships. Unburden me
by listening to my sins and by forgiving me.
Hold me, Jesus, and comfort me. Help me to
always believe that you are with me and will not
abandon me. Help me to always trust in your
unconditional love for me. Thank you, O God,
for helping me in my cancer illness.
Amen.

May the God of life be with you, calming your
fears and teaching you to trust in his gracious
love and mercy. May you be strengthened for
your fight, and guided to choices for healing
and wholeness. And may you be filled with joy
and peace in experiencing God's presence on
your journey.
Amen.

☙

– Jeanne's Epilogue –

O LORD, you have searched me and known
me. I praise you, for I am fearfully and
wonderfully made. Wonderful
are your works; that I know very well.

PSALM 139:1, 14

The week between my CT scan and MRI on March 22, 2001, and my doctor's appointment on March 28—in which I would receive the results—was very ordinary and calm. I had told everyone I knew to pray for me before the tests, and now I had a week's reprieve before I had to face the news. I often daydreamed about hearing that my tumors were gone and about what it would be like to shout my good news from the rooftops. On the day of the doctor's appointment, I prayed with friends—as well as with my husband in the doctor's waiting room—for me to feel God's peace and presence with me no matter the results.

When Dr. Denes knocked on the door, I told him only to come in if he had good news. He said he did. I think I stopped breathing until I listened to him say that many of my tumors were smaller. I jumped up and danced around in the examining room, hugging my doctor and my husband. I had never had a reduction in my tumors. Now, for the first time, I had tumors appear smaller in size; I had no new tumors; and, to the amazement of everyone, the three tumors around my pancreas were no longer there.

Easter came early for me this year! I have been shouting my good news from the rooftops and praising and thanking God. The first thing I thought was how wonderful it will be to dance at our daughter's wedding next summer. Now when we shop for her wedding dress, I can daydream about seeing her walk down the aisle in it. It seems so unreal to actually have good news. For the past five years, the most I could say was, "No major growth or spread," major being the key word, in that it always meant at least some growth in my tumors.

During one of the happy phone calls to an old friend, I detailed all the tumor changes in my lungs, chest, kidney, and pancreas. Then I stated, "God is so good! Thank you for your prayers." Her response helped put things in perspective. She said, "Either way; even if your cancer had gotten worse, God is still good." I told her she was right. I prayed for God's peace and presence, no matter what. And I continue to trust in God's goodness to mend my family, whether this reduction continues or not. My gratitude now is as much for the love and support I feel from God being with me, as it is for the reduction in my tumors. Either way it ends up, God is indeed good!

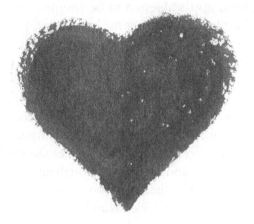

– Linda's Epilogue –

ॐ

When you come to the edge of all the light
you know and are about to step off into the
darkness of the unknown, faith is knowing one
of two things will happen: there will be something solid to stand on or you will be taught
how to fly.

Barbara J. Winter

I am proud and so blessed to be Jeanne's twin sister and also blessed to call her my best friend. It is truly a privilege and a grace to write this final chapter in Jeanne's book.

In January 2002 Jeanne was diagnosed with four brain tumors. Her only option for survival was whole-brain radiation. Jeanne underwent three weeks of the radiation treatments. She was extremely fatigued due to the treatments, so much so that at times she could not tie her own shoes and barely had enough energy to walk from her bedroom to the family room. Jeanne's husband, Tom, took off work, and friends and family continued to give Jeanne hope and support and to pray unceasingly. Jeanne seemed to regain her energy little by little, and that following July Jeanne and Tom walked their daughter, Debbie, down the aisle at her wedding.

I accompanied Jeanne to the Bahamas for her alternative cancer treatment shortly after the wedding. While we were there, Jeanne's husband, Tom, called with the news that her latest scans showed that the brain tumors were not growing. Jeanne was ecstatic and filled with hope. September 2002 brought the birth of a new grandson. In October, Jeanne was dancing at my daughter's wedding. It seemed that she beat the odds once again.

In January 2003, tests revealed that one of the brain tumors seemed to be growing, so Jeanne underwent Gamma-Knife surgery. The brain tumors held their own but the nodules in Jeanne's lungs were growing and causing a great deal of coughing and difficulty taking deep breaths. Jeanne had two thoracic surgeries in August to help make it easier for her to breathe. She had a tumor in her windpipe that was cutting off the air to the third lobe of her right lung. Jeanne fractured ribs with all of her coughing.

On Christmas 2003, Jeanne insisted on hosting our family celebration because she said she couldn't let the cancer win. Another new grandson was welcomed into the family after Christmas.

The doctors wanted to schedule another broncho-scope for the beginning of January 2004 to open Jeanne's airways to make her breathing easier, but Jeanne had other plans. She had been asked to be part of the team on a girls' senior high school retreat. Jeanne cared very deeply about the girls' personal relationship with God and believed in the retreat's message of God's passionate love for each of us. Jeanne was determined to make the retreat and give her talk. At this point it was difficult for Jeanne to breathe and speak at the same time. It was certainly with the grace of God that Jeanne was able to present her talk titled, "Obstacles to God's Friendship." Jeanne shared with the girls that sometimes our choices get in the way of receiving God's love. She shared her fears and her struggles, how she felt powerless and weak when she heard the latest test results. She shared that sometimes she acted how she thought her family and friends expected her to act. She wanted to live up to their expectations. She wore the mask of a "rock" to protect those she loved and herself. This was her coping mechanism. She was expected to be a rock, a fighter, to be positive and an inspiration to others. And so she was—wearing the mask of a rock. She wanted to protect her family and loved ones; she could worry enough for all of them. Jeanne was afraid of others' rejection and pity. Jeanne shared with the girls that she knew she could not wear a mask that could hide the real her from Jesus who knew her and was walking with her. Jeanne shared that she was finding strength in Jesus' friendship through her husband, daughters, and sisters.

It was so important to Jeanne to tell the girls about God's faithfulness and intimate love for each of them. Jeanne told the girls that God accepts us for who we are and that Jesus gives each of us the strength we need in our weaknesses to be ourselves.

> (The Lord) said to me, "My grace is sufficient for you, for power is made perfect in weakness." So, I will boast all the more gladly of my weaknesses, so that the power of Christ may dwell in me. Therefore I am content with weaknesses, insults, hardships, persecutions, and calamities for the sake of Christ; for whenever I am weak, then I am strong.
>
> 2 Corinthians 12:9–(10

While Jeanne was on that January retreat, her daughter, Barbara, and her fiancé entered a contest to win a mega-wedding sponsored by a local radio station. The original date of the wedding was set for May of that year. Barbara and David entered the contest because Barbara wanted both her parents to walk her down the aisle, and she knew Jeanne's health was failing. Barbara and Dave won the mega-wedding which was scheduled for February 13.

Just three weeks after that retreat Jeanne went into the hospital. Six days later Jeanne died peacefully, surrounded by her family, on February 8, 2004. We have no doubt that Jesus was right there welcoming Jeanne into his eternal life with a big hug. The day before Jeanne died, Barbara got her wish for her mom to be at her wedding. Barbara and David exchanged their vows in the ICU room before a priest and many family members.

After Jeanne died, someone called our attention to the roses next to Jeanne's bed. There were five red roses, one each for Tom, Jeanne, and their three daughters. There were also four white roses, one for each of the three sons-in-law, and one for Jesus. The head of one of the red roses was bent over. No one had noticed it like that before Jeanne died.

Two years after Jeanne died, a new grandson was born on the anniversary of Jeanne's death. Life on earth ends; life begins. We are to celebrate life—this life on earth and new life in eternity.

Saint Irenaeus is credited with saying that the glory of God is a person fully alive. Jeanne's life and almost twenty-year battle with cancer gave God great glory. All who love Jeanne continue to carry her in our hearts and in all we do. Jeanne and her story are ongoing. Jeanne continues to do what she did best—inspire, challenge, and invite people to a change of heart in order to experience God's love and mercy in the midst of both pain and joy. Death is a reality of life, and we cannot escape it. Jeanne did not lose the battle with cancer; she won it, living for nearly twenty years after the original diagnosis, by living with such dignity and grace, and by living her faith with an incredible spirit. The more difficult her struggle became, the more she looked to Jesus for strength and hope.

May all who read Jeanne's journey about facing cancer with God's help—no matter what struggles and difficulties may be before you—be filled with a renewed belief in the sacredness of life, God's faithfulness, mercy and intimate love. And may you be filled with hope in the power of the resurrection. God is good. God is indeed good.

꿎

I am already being poured out as a libation,
and the time of my departure has come. I have
fought the good fight, I have finished the race,
I have kept the faith. From now on there is
reserved for me the crown of righteousness,
which the Lord, the righteous judge, will give
me on that day, and not only to me but also
to all who have longed for his appearing.
But the Lord stood by me and gave me strength,
so that through me the message might be fully
proclaimed and all the Gentiles might hear it.
So I was rescued from the lion's mouth. The
Lord will rescue me from every evil attack and
save me for his heavenly kingdom. To him be
the glory forever and ever. Amen.

2 TIMOTHY 4:6–8, 17–18

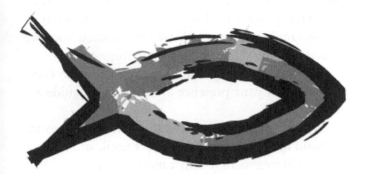

– Appendix A –
Prayers for Healing and Hope

෩

Death is not extinguishing the light; it is putting
out the lamp because the Dawn has come.

RABINDRANATH TAGORE

PRAYER FOR FIGHTING CANCER

Lord, I am frightened at my diagnosis of cancer. How will I handle all the decisions that must be made? How will my family and I cope? Dear Jesus, I know you love me and that you will never abandon me.

Give me the strength and courage I need to cope. Bless me with your presence and peace, and guide my every decision.

Walk with my family and let them know you are with me. Send me the support and help I need, and lead me to the right treatment for my cancer.

Let your angels guard me and keep me pointed in the right direction. I offer my suffering to you and unite it with your pain and suffering on the cross. May good come out of this time of crisis in my life.

Help me to forgive those who need my forgiveness, and help me to seek forgiveness from those I've hurt. Help me to make loving choices and to be a witness of your love to all I meet on this cancer journey. Hold me, Lord. And walk with me every step on this journey. Amen.

෫ல

PRAYER BEFORE AN OPERATION

Dear Creator God, I come to you with all my fears as I face this surgery. Please give me the courage I need to face the day with steady confidence in your protection and love. When I am in the deep sleep needed for the operation, give assurance to my spirit within that I need not worry or be afraid. Calm my nerves, put my mind at ease, and, in your mercy, forgive me all my sins.

Please give the medical team the required skills needed to perform successful surgery with no complications. Please give my family and friends the reassuring faith that you are with us. Calm all their anxieties during the coming hours of my operation.

I place my recovery in your hands and ask for your healing touch to speed my return to health.

Dear God, I place my life in your hands and trust in your goodness, care, and love for me. I ask you to hear me in the name of Jesus, your Son. Amen.

ৎৡ

PRAYER FOR CHEMOTHERAPY

Loving God, you are the source of my strength. I come to you now as I begin my chemotherapy treatment. Please guide these drugs to seek and destroy all cancer cells, and protect my healthy cells from harm. Send your healing power to my body so that I will have little or no adverse effects from the treatment. Help my stomach to be strong and not to be nauseous. Give me your energy and save me from fatigue. If possible, let me keep both my good spirits and my hair. Dear God, I know you love me so much. Please help me to hold up under this treatment, with faith and trust in your protective arms. No matter the effects, I trust your healing love to hold me and comfort me. Amen.

PRAYER FOR RADIATION THERAPY

Good and gracious God, you continue to be my source of strength. I come to you now as I begin my radiation therapy. Please bless all who will attend to me, that their skill in directing the radiation will be successful. Guide the rays, that all the cancer cells will be eradicated and all my healthy cells will be protected from harm.

Send your healing power to my body so that I will have little or no adverse affects from the treatment.

I know you love me so much. Please help me to endure this treatment with faith and trust. No matter the effects, I trust your healing love to hold me and comfort me. Amen.

❧

PRAYER FOR RELIEF OF PAIN

Lord Jesus, you certainly knew pain. Please be present with me as I endure my suffering. If possible, take this pain away, and let me feel your peace and comfort throughout my body and in my mind and heart as well. I ask for relief, even if only for a short while. Give me your strength and allow me to feel your love and follow your example. I offer up my pain for this special intention (name it). I love you and need you today and always. Amen.

PRAYER FOR WHEN I WANT TO GIVE UP

Dear Jesus, I am so weary and tired of the fight. At times, I just want to give up. I wish you could just hold me and tell me it's going to be alright. I don't like feeling so weak and sick. I'm tired of asking people to wait on me, and help me because I cannot take care of my own needs.

I need you now, Lord, to replace my weakness with your strength, to replace my doubts with faith in your care for me, and to replace my fears with your love for me. Send me your Spirit, that I may wake up tomorrow, feeling and knowing you are with me, and that I can go on.

I trust you, Lord, to tell me when it's time to stop the fight to hang on to this mortal life. Bless every moment of my life with goodness and kindness and peace. And bless my transition with peace and joy when I pass to the new life that awaits me in heaven. Amen.

⚘

PSALM 23: THE LORD IS MY SHEPHERD

The Lord is my shepherd, I shall not want.
He makes me lie down in green pastures;
he leads me beside still waters;
he restores my soul.
He leads me in right paths for his name's sake.
Even though I walk through the darkest valley,
I fear no evil; for you are with me;
your rod and your staff—they comfort me.

107

You prepare a table before me in the presence
of my enemies; you anoint my head with oil;
my cup overflows.
Surely goodness and mercy shall follow me
all the days of my life, and I shall dwell in the
house of the Lord my whole life long.

ANIMA CHRISTI

Soul of Christ, sanctify me
Body of Christ, save me
Blood of Christ, inebriate me
Water from Christ's side, wash me
Passion of Christ, strengthen me
O good Jesus, hear me
Within Thy wounds hide me
Suffer me not to be separated from Thee
From the malicious enemy defend me
In the hour of my death call me
And bid me come unto Thee
That I may praise Thee with Thy saints
and with Thy angels
Forever and ever
Amen.

THE TANDEM BIKE RIDE

At first, I saw God as my observer, my judge—keeping track of things I did to know whether I merited heaven or hell. God was "out there"—sort of like a president: I recognized his picture, but I did not know him.

Later on, when I met Jesus, life became a bike ride. It was a tandem bike, and Jesus was in the back helping me pedal. I don't know at what point he suggested we change places, but life has not been the same since then.

When I had the control, I knew the way. It was rather boring, but predictable. It was the shortest distance between two points. When Jesus led, we took delightful long cuts—up mountains and through rocky places at breakneck speeds. It was all I could do to hang on! Even though it looked like madness, he said, "Pedal!" I worried and was anxious and asked, "Where are you taking me?" He laughed, but didn't answer.

I forgot my boring life and entered into the adventure. And when I would say, "I'm scared," he'd lean back and touch my hand. He took me to people who gave me gifts of healing, acceptance, joy, and peace for our journey. He said, "Give the gifts away." So I did—to the people we met. And I found that in giving I received, and our burden was light.

I did not trust him at first to control my life. I thought he'd wreck it. But he knows how to make bikes bend and take sharp corners, jump to clear high rocks, fly to shorten scary passages.

I am learning to be quiet and pedal in the strangest places. I'm beginning to enjoy the view and the cool breeze on my face.

And when I'm sure I just can't do any more, he just smiles and says, "Pedal!"

ANONYMOUS

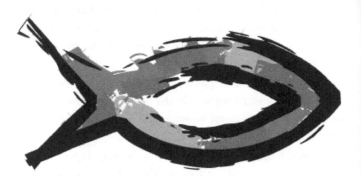

– Appendix B –

Recommended Books

℘

I am listing some of the books that have been most helpful to me. You can borrow them from the library, hospital cancer-support centers, or local cancer-support organizations. Some books are also available in DVD or CD format.

PRAYER/HOPE SUPPORT

Joan Wester Anderson, *Where Angels Walk* (New York: Simon & Schuster, 1994).

Joan Wester Anderson, *An Angel to Watch Over Me: True Stories of Children's Encounters With Angels* (New York: Ballantine, 1994).

Joan Wester Anderson, *Where Miracles Happen: True Stories of Angel Encounters* (Loyola Press, 2009).

Jack Canfield, *Chicken Soup for the Soul: 101 Stories to Open the Heart and Rekindle the Spirit* (Backlist LLC, 2012).

Yitaa Halberstam, and Judith Leventhal, *Small Miracles* (Holbrook, MA: Adams Media, 1997).

Harold S. Kushner, *When Bad Things Happen to Good People* (New York: Anchor, 2004).

Thomas Merton, *Contemplative Prayer* (Garden City, NY: Doubleday, 1980).

Fr. Seraphim Michalenko, MIC, *The Divine Mercy Message and Devotion* (Stockbridge, MA: Marian Helpers, 1995).

Diana Losciale, *Prayers for Coping With Cancer: Making the Journey* (Liguori, MO, Liguori Publications, 2009).

Basil Pennington, *Centering Prayer* (Garden City, NY: Doubleday, 1980).

The Story of Fatima is told in a booklet published by the Mother of Christ Crusade, Inc., 1444 Janie Ave., Billings, Montana 59101. Published in 1947.

৵৯

AFTERLIFE

Maggie Callanan and Patricia Kelley, *Final Gifts* (New York: Simon and Schuster, 2012).

Raymond Moody, *Reflections on Life After Life* (New York: Bantam, 1978).

Peter Shockey, *Reflections of Heaven* (New York: Doubleday, 1999).

Brad Steiger, *One With the Light* (New York: Signet, 1994).

ൠ

MIND/BODY/SPIRIT TREATMENT AND SUPPORT:

Bernie Siegel, *Love, Medicine & Miracles* (New York: Harper, 1990).

Bernie Siegel, *Peace, Love & Healing* (New York: Harper, 1990).

Carl Simonton, *Getting Well Again* (New York: Bantam Books, 1992).

Joan Borysenko, *Minding the Body, Mending the Mind* (DeCapo Press, 2007).

Andrew Weil, *Spontaneous Healing* (Ballantine Books, 2000).

Andrew Weil, *Eight Weeks to Optimum Health* (New York: Ballantine Books, 2007).

ൠ

GRIEF

Martha Whitmore Hickman, *Healing After Loss: A Daily Journal for Working Through Grief* (Peter Pauper Press, 2012).

Doveen, *How to Heal a Grieving Heart* (Hay House, 2013).

Gretchen Schwenker, *Every Tear Will be Wiped Away: Prayers for Comfort in Times of Grief* (Liguori Publications, 2011).

CPSIA information can be obtained at www.ICGtesting.com
Printed in the USA
LVOW05s1032290914

406347LV00001B/1/P